Cardiac, Chest, Airway, and Respiratory Impairment

Identification, Management, and Treatment of Diseases and Injuries

Subcourses MD0568, MD0569, and MD0571

Edition 100

Cardiac, Chest, Airway, and Respiratory Impairment

Identification, Management, and Treatment of Diseases and Injuries

Subcourses MD0568, MD0569, and MD0571

Edition 100

Cardiac, Chest, Airway, and Respiratory Impairment: Identification, Management, and Treatment of Diseases and Injuries

PharmaLogika, Inc.
PO Box 461
Willow Springs, NC 27592

www.pharmalogika.com

Author / Editor: Mindy J. Allport-Settle

Published by PharmaLogika, Inc.

Printed in the United States of America.

ISBN 1-9372580-6-8
ISBN-13 978-1-937258-06-1

Contents

Overview **1**
About this Book 1
Included Documents and Features 1

Introduction **3**
Cardiopulmonary (Circulatory) System 3
Human Cardiovascular System 3
Pulmonary Circulation 4
Systemic Circulation 4
Coronary Circulation 4
Heart 4
Closed Cardiovascular System 5
Oxygen Transportation 5
Development 5
Arterial Development 5
Venous Development 6
Measurement Techniques 6
Human Lung 6
Anatomy 7
Human Lungs 8
Modification of Substances 9
Non respiratory functions 9
Army Medical Command 11
Structure and Subordinate Commands 11
Operations 12
In Garrison (Peacetime) 12
Deployments 12
Army Medical Department 12
Medical Special Branches 13
United States Army Training and Doctrine Command 13
TRADOC History 14
TRADOC Priorities 15

Respiratory Diseases and Disorders

Introduction

1. Anatomy and Physiology of the Respiratory System

Section I. Structure and Function of the Respiratory Organs 1-1

Section II. Accessory Structures of the Respiratory System ... 1-6
Section III. Physiology of Respiration 1-10
Exercises

2. Physical Assessment of the Respiratory System
Section I. General Approach to Physical Assessment 2-1
Section II. Steps of the Procedure 2-5
Exercises

3. Infectious Respiratory Diseases
Section I. Upper Respiratory Diseases 3-1
Section II. Upper Respiratory Diseases with Systemic Effects 3-6
Section III. Lower Respiratory Diseases 3-8
Section IV. Other Causes of Pneumonia 3-11
Exercises

4. Chronic Obstructive Pulmonary Diseases
Section I. Asthma 4-1
Section II. Chronic Bronchitis 4-5
Section III. Emphysema 4-8
Exercises

5. Respiratory Disorders
Section I. Hyperventilation Syndrome 5-1
Section II. Spontaneous Pneumothorax 5-4
Section III. Pulmonary Embolism 5-8
Section IV. Inhaled Toxic Substances 5-13
Exercises

6. Tuberculosis 6-1
Exercises

Chest and Airway Problems

Introduction

1. Chest Trauma

Section I. General Information About Chest injuries 1-1

Section II. Specific Chest Injuries 1-6

Section III. Chest Decompression 1-14

Exercises

2. Airway Management

Section I. Esophageal Obturator Airway 2-1

Section II. Endotracheal Tube 2-7

Exercises

3. Cricothyroidotomy

Section I. General Considerations 3-1

Section II. Needle Cricothyroidotomy 3-5

Section III. Surgical Cricothyroidotomy 3-7

Exercises

Cardiac Impairment

Introduction

1. Basic Cardiac Life Support

Section I. General Information 1-1

Section II. Rescue Breathing 1-8

Section III. Chest Compressions 1-10

Section IV. One-Rescuer Method CPR 1-13

Section V. Two-Rescuer Method CPR 1-15

Section VI. CPR Complications/CPR Termination 1-21

Exercises

2. Dysrhythmia Recognition and Treatment

Section I. Dysrhythmia 2-1

Section II. Electrophysiology 2-3

Section III. Rhythms/Heart Blocks 2-6

Exercises

3. Cardiac Arrest (Defibrillation)

Section I. Review of the Cardiovascular System and the Respiratory System 3-1

Section II. General Considerations Regarding Cardiac Arrest 3-6

Section III. Major Management Techniques of Cardiac Arrest 3-11

Section IV. Cardioversion 3-15

Overview

About this Book

The United States Army is recognized internationally as the standard for complete, efficient and effective adult education. The Army has a tradition of pioneering training systems (including computer-based training) that then transition into the civilian corporate sector.

This manual has been continuously tested and updated to successfully educate every member of the modern United States Army. The needs of the instructor, the student, and the Army are perfectly balanced. This is the model all educators strive to follow when developing and delivering training programs.

Included Documents and Features

Respiratory Diseases and Disorders

1. Anatomy and Physiology of the Respiratory System
2. Physical Assessment of the Respiratory System
3. Infectious Respiratory Diseases
4. Chronic Obstructive Pulmonary Diseases
5. Respiratory Disorders
6. Tuberculosis

Chest and Airway Problems

1. Chest Trauma
2. Airway Management
3. Cricothyroidotomy

Cardiac Impairment

1. Basic Cardiac Life Support
2. Dysrhythmia Recognition and Treatment
3. Cardiac Arrest (Defibrillation)

Exercises Supporting Each Section

Introduction

Cardiopulmonary (Circulatory) System

The circulatory system is an organ system that passes nutrients (such as amino acids, electrolytes and lymph), gases, hormones, blood cells, etc. to and from cells in the body to help fight diseases, stabilize body temperature and pH, and to maintain homeostasis.

This system may be seen strictly as a blood distribution network, but some consider the circulatory system as composed of the cardiovascular system, which distributes blood[1], and the lymphatic system[2], which distributes lymph. While humans, as well as other vertebrates, have a closed cardiovascular system (meaning that the blood never leaves the network of arteries, veins and capillaries), some invertebrate groups have an open cardiovascular system. The most primitive animal phyla lack circulatory systems. The lymphatic system, on the other hand, is an open system.

Two types of fluids move through the circulatory system: blood and lymph. The blood, heart, and blood vessels form the cardiovascular system. The lymph, lymph nodes, and lymph vessels form the lymphatic system. The cardiovascular system and the lymphatic system collectively make up the circulatory system.

Human Cardiovascular System

The main components of the human cardiovascular system are the heart, blood, and blood vessels[3]. It includes: the pulmonary circulation, a "loop" through the lungs where blood is oxygenated; and the systemic circulation, a "loop" through the rest of the body to provide oxygenated blood. An average adult contains five to six quarts (roughly 4.7 to 5.7 liters) of blood, which consists of plasma, red blood cells, white blood cells, and platelets. Also, the digestive system works with the circulatory system to provide the nutrients the system needs to keep the heart pumping.

---

[1] "Cardiovascular system" at Dorland's Medical Dictionary

[2] "Lymphatic system" at Dorland's Medical Dictionary

[3] National Library of Medicine MeSH classification

Pulmonary Circulation

The pulmonary circulatory system is the portion of the cardiovascular system in which oxygen-depleted blood is pumped away from the heart, via the pulmonary artery, to the lungs and returned, oxygenated, to the heart via the pulmonary vein.

Oxygen deprived blood from the vena cava, enters the right atrium of the heart and flows through the tricuspid valve (right atrioventricular valve) into the right ventricle, from which it is then pumped through the pulmonary semilunar valve into the pulmonary artery to the lungs. Gas exchange occurs in the lungs, whereby CO2 is released from the blood, and oxygen is absorbed. The pulmonary vein returns the now oxygen-rich blood to the heart.

Systemic Circulation

Systemic circulation is the portion of the cardiovascular system which transports oxygenated blood away from the heart, to the rest of the body, and returns oxygen-depleted blood back to the heart. Systemic circulation is, distance-wise, much longer than pulmonary circulation, transporting blood to every part of the body.

Coronary Circulation

The coronary circulatory system provides a blood supply to the heart. As it provides oxygenated blood to the heart, it is by definition a part of the systemic circulatory system.

Heart

The heart pumps oxygenated blood to the body and deoxygenated blood to the lungs. In the human heart there is one atrium and one ventricle for each circulation, and with both a systemic and a pulmonary circulation there are four chambers in total: left atrium, left ventricle, right atrium and right ventricle. The right atrium is the upper chamber of the right side of the heart. The blood that is returned to the right atrium is deoxygenated (poor in oxygen) and passed into the right ventricle to be pumped through the pulmonary artery to the lungs for re-oxygenation and removal of carbon dioxide. The left atrium receives newly oxygenated blood from the lungs as well as the pulmonary vein which is passed into the strong left ventricle to be pumped through the aorta to the different organs of the body.

Closed Cardiovascular System

The cardiovascular systems of humans are closed, meaning that the blood never leaves the network of blood vessels. In contrast, oxygen and nutrients diffuse across the blood vessel layers and enters interstitial fluid, which carries oxygen and nutrients to the target cells, and carbon dioxide and wastes in the opposite direction. The other component of the circulatory system, the lymphatic system, is not closed.

Oxygen Transportation

About 98.5% of the oxygen in a sample of arterial blood in a healthy human breathing air at sea-level pressure is chemically combined with haemoglobin molecules. About 1.5% is physically dissolved in the other blood liquids and not connected to haemoglobin. The haemoglobin molecule is the primary transporter of oxygen in mammals and many other species.

Development

The development of the circulatory system initially occurs by the process of vasculogenesis. The human arterial and venous systems develop from different embryonic areas. While the arterial system develops mainly from the aortic arches, the venous system arises from three bilateral veins during weeks 4 - 8 of human development.

Arterial Development

The human arterial system originate from the aortic arches and from the dorsal aortae starting from week 4 of human development. Aortic arch 1 almost completely regresses except to form the maxillary arteries. Aortic arch 2 also completely regresses except to form the stapedial arteries. The definitive formation of the arterial system arise from aortic arches 3, 4 and 6. While aortic arch 5 completely regreses.

The dorsal aortae are initially bilateral and then fuse to form the definitive dorsal aorta. Approximately 30 posterolateral branches arise off the aorta and will form the intercostal arteries, upper and lower extremity arteries, lumbar arteries and the lateral sacral arteries. The lateral branches of the aorta form the definitive renal, suprarrenal and gonadal arteries. Finally, the ventral branches of the aorta consist of the vitelline arteries and umbilical arteries. The vitelline arteries form the celiac, superior and inferior mesenteric arteries of the gastrointestinal tract. After birth, the umbilical arteries will form the internal iliac arteries.

Venous Development

The human venous system develops mainly from the vitelline veins, the umbilical veins and the cardinal veins, all of which empty into the sinus venosus.

Measurement Techniques

- Electrocardiogram—for cardiac electrophysiology
- Sphygmomanometer and stethoscope—for blood pressure
- Pulse meter—for cardiac function (heart rate, rhythm, dropped beats)
- Pulse—commonly used to determine the heart rate in absence of certain cardiac pathologies
- Heart rate variability -- used to measure variations of time intervals between heart beats
- Nail bed blanching test—test for perfusion
- Vessel cannula or catheter pressure measurement—pulmonary wedge pressure or in older animal experiments.

Human Lung

The lungs of mammals have a spongelike and soft texture and are honeycombed with epithelium, having a much larger surface area in total than the outer surface area of the lung itself. The lungs of humans are a typical example of this type of lung.

Breathing is largely driven by the muscular diaphragm at the bottom of the thorax. Contraction of the diaphragm pulls the bottom of the cavity in which the lung is enclosed downward, increasing volume and thus decreasing pressure, causing air to flow into the airways. Air enters through the oral and nasal cavities; it flows through the pharynx, then the larynx and into the trachea, which branches out into the main bronchi and then subsequent divisions. During normal breathing, expiration is passive and no muscles are contracted (the diaphragm relaxes). The rib cage itself is also able to expand and contract to some degree, through the action of other respiratory and accessory respiratory muscles. As a result, air is transported into or expelled out of the lungs. This type of lung is known as a bellows lung as it resembles a blacksmith's bellows.[4]

The human lungs are the organs of respiration in humans. Humans have two lungs. Together, the lungs contain approximately 2,400 kilometres (1,500 mi) of airways and 300 to 500 million alveoli, having a total surface area of about 70 square metres (750 sq ft) (8,4 x 8,4 m) in adults — roughly the same area as one side of a tennis court[5]. Furthermore, if all of the capillaries that surround the alveoli were unwound and laid end to end, they would extend for about 992 kilometres (616 mi). Each lung weighs 1.1 kilograms (2.4 lb), therefore making the entire organ about 2.3 kilograms (5.1 lb).

Anatomy

In humans, the trachea divides into the two main bronchi that enter the roots of the lungs. The bronchi continue to divide within the lung, and after multiple divisions, give rise to bronchioles. The bronchial tree continues branching until it reaches the level of terminal bronchioles, which lead to alveolar sacs. Alveolar sacs are made up of clusters of alveoli, like individual grapes within a bunch. The individual alveoli are tightly wrapped in blood vessels and it is here that gas exchange actually occurs. Deoxygenated blood from the heart is pumped through the pulmonary artery to the lungs, where oxygen diffuses into blood and is exchanged for carbon dioxide in the hemoglobin of the erythrocytes. The oxygen-rich blood returns to the heart via the pulmonary veins to be pumped back into systemic circulation.

Human lungs are located in two cavities on either side of the heart. Though similar in appearance, the two are not identical. Both are separated into lobes by fissures, with three lobes on the right and two on the left. The lobes are further divided into segments and then into lobules, hexagonal divisions of the lungs that are the smallest subdivision visible to the naked eye. The connective tissue that divides lobules is often blackened in smokers. The medial border of the right lung is nearly vertical, while the left lung contains a cardiac notch. The cardiac notch is a concave impression molded to accommodate the shape of the heart.

Each lobe is surrounded by a pleural cavity, which consists of two pleurae. The parietal pleura lies against the rib cage, and the visceral pleura lies on the surface of the lungs. In between the pleura is pleural fluid. The pleural cavity helps the

---

[4] Maton, Anthea; Jean Hopkins, Charles William McLaughlin, Susan Johnson, Maryanna Quon Warner, David LaHart, Jill D. Wright1 (1993). Human Biology and Health. Englewood Cliffs, New Jersey, USA: Prentice Hall. ISBN 0-13-981176-1. OCLC 32308337.

[5] Notter, Robert H. (2000). *Lung surfactants: basic science and clinical applications.* New York, N.Y: Marcel Dekker. pp. 120. ISBN 0-8247-0401-0. Retrieved 2008-10-11.

lubricate the lungs, as well as providing surface tension to keep the lung surface in contact with the rib cage.

Lungs are to a certain extent 'overbuilt' and have a tremendous reserve volume as compared to the oxygen exchange requirements when at rest. Such excess capacity is one of the reasons that individuals can smoke for years without having a noticeable decrease in lung function while still or moving slowly; in situations like these only a small portion of the lungs are actually perfused with blood for gas exchange. Destruction of too many alveoli over time leads to the condition emphysema, which is associated with extreme shortness of breath. As oxygen requirements increase due to exercise, a greater volume of the lungs is perfused, allowing the body to match its CO_2/O_2 exchange requirements. Additionally, due to the excess capacity, it is possible for humans to live with only one lung, with the one compensating for the other's loss.

The environment of the lung is very moist, which makes it hospitable for bacteria. Many respiratory illnesses are the result of bacterial or viral infection of the lungs. Inflammation of the lungs is known as pneumonia; inflammation of the pleura surrounding the lungs is known as pleurisy.

Vital capacity is the maximum volume of air that a person can exhale after maximum inhalation; it can be measured with a spirometer. In combination with other physiological measurements, the vital capacity can help make a diagnosis of underlying lung disease.

The lung parenchyma is strictly used to refer solely to alveolar tissue with respiratory bronchioles, alveolar ducts and terminal bronchioles. However, it often includes any form of lung tissue, also including bronchioles, bronchi, blood vessels and lung interstitium.[6]

Human Lungs

The conducting zone contains the trachea, the bronchi, the bronchioles, and the terminal bronchioles The respiratory zone contains the respiratory bronchioles, the alveolar ducts, and the alveoli. The conducting zone and the respiratory stuffers (but not the alveoli) are made up of airways. The conducting zone has no gas exchange with the blood, and is reinforced with cartilage in order to hold open the airways. The conducting zone warms the air to 37 °C (99 °F) and humidifies the air. It also cleanses the air by removing particles via cilia located on the walls of all the passageways. The lungs are surrounded by the rib cage. The respiratory zone is the site of gas exchange with blood.

[6] Medilexicon.com > Medical Dictionary – 'Parenchyma Of Lung' In turn citing: Stedman's Medical Dictionary. 2006.

- The sympathetic nervous system via noradrenaline acting on the beta receptors causes bronchodilation.

- The parasympathetic nervous system via acetylcholine, which acts on the M-1 muscarinic receptors, maintains the resting tone of the bronchiolar smooth muscle. This action is related, although considered distinct from bronchoconstriction.

- Many other non-autonomic nervous and biochemical stimuli, including carbon dioxide and oxygen, are also involved in the regulation process.

The pleural cavity is the potential space between the parietal pleura, lining the inner wall of the thoracic cage, and the visceral pleura lining the lungs.

The lung parenchyma is strictly used to refer solely to alveolar tissue with respiratory bronchioles, alveolar ducts and terminal bronchioles. However, it often includes any form of lung tissue, also including bronchioles, bronchi, blood vessels and lung interstitium[7].

Modification of Substances

The lungs convert angiotensin I to angiotensin II. In addition, they remove several blood-borne substances, e.g. PGE1, PGE2, PGF2α, leukotrienes, serotonin, bradykinin[8].

Non respiratory functions

In addition to their function in respiration, the lungs also:

- Alter the pH of blood by facilitating alterations in the partial pressure of carbon dioxide

- Filter out small blood clots formed in veins

- Filter out gas micro-bubbles occurring in the venous blood stream such as those created during decompression after underwater diving.[9]

- Influence the concentration of some biologic substances and drugs used in medicine in blood

[7] Medilexicon.com > Medical Dictionary – 'Parenchyma Of Lung' In turn citing: Stedman's Medical Dictionary. 2006.
[8] Walter F., PhD. Boron (2004). Medical Physiology: A Cellular And Molecular Approaoch. Elsevier/Saunders. ISBN 1-4160-2328-3. Page 605.
[9] Wienke B.R. : "Decompression theory."

- Convert angiotensin I to angiotensin II by the action of angiotensin-converting enzyme

- May serve as a layer of soft, shock-absorbent protection for the heart, which the lungs flank and nearly enclose.

- Immunoglobulin-A is secreted in the bronchial secretion and protects against respiratory infections.

- Maintain sterility by producing mucus containing antimicrobial compounds.[10] Mucus contains glycoproteins, e.g. mucins, lactoferrin,[11] lysozyme, lactoperoxidase.[12, 13] We find also on the epithelium Dual oxidase 2[14, 15, 16] proteins generating hydrogen peroxide, useful for hypothiocyanite endogenous antimicrobial synthesis. Function not in place in cystic fibrosis patient lungs.[17, 18]

- Ciliary escalator action is an important defence system against air-borne infection.The dust particles and bacteria in the inhaled air are caught in the mucous layer present at the mucosal surface of respiratory passages and are moved up towards pharynx by the rhythmic upward beating action of the cilia.

---

[10] Travis SM, Conway BA, Zabner J, et al. (May 1999). "Activity of abundant antimicrobials of the human airway." American Journal of Respiratory Cell and Molecular Biology 20 (5): 872–9.
[11] Rogan MP, Taggart CC, Greene CM, Murphy PG, O'Neill SJ, McElvaney NG (October 2004). "Loss of microbicidal activity and increased formation of biofilm due to decreased lactoferrin activity in patients with cystic fibrosis". The Journal of Infectious Diseases 190 (7): 1245–53.
[12] Wijkstrom-Frei C, El-Chemaly S, Ali-Rachedi R, et al. (August 2003). "Lactoperoxidase and human airway host defense". American Journal of Respiratory Cell and Molecular Biology 29 (2): 206–12.
[13] Conner GE, Salathe M, Forteza R (December 2002). "Lactoperoxidase and hydrogen peroxide metabolism in the airway". American Journal of Respiratory and Critical Care Medicine 166 (12 Pt 2): S57–61.
[14] Fischer H (October 2009). "Mechanisms and Function of DUOX in Epithelia of the Lung". Antioxidants & Redox Signaling 11 (10): 2453–65.
[15] Rada B, Leto TL (2008). "Oxidative innate immune defenses by Nox/Duox family NADPH Oxidases." Contributions to Microbiology. Contributions to Microbiology 15: 164–87.
[16] Rada B, Lekstrom K, Damian S, Dupuy C, Leto TL (October 2008). "The Pseudomonas toxin pyocyanin inhibits the Dual oxidase-based antimicrobial system as it imposes oxidative stress on airway epithelial cells". Journal of Immunology 181 (7): 4883–93.
[17] Moskwa P, Lorentzen D, Excoffon KJ, et al. (January 2007). "A Novel Host Defense System of Airways Is Defective in Cystic Fibrosis". American Journal of Respiratory and Critical Care Medicine 175 (2): 174–83.
[18] Conner GE, Wijkstrom-Frei C, Randell SH, Fernandez VE, Salathe M (January 2007). "The Lactoperoxidase System Links Anion Transport To Host Defense in Cystic Fibrosis". FEBS Letters 581 (2): 271–8.

- Provide airflow for the creation of vocal sounds.
- Thermoregulation (panting)

Army Medical Command

The U.S. Army Medical Command (MEDCOM) is a major command of the U.S. Army that provides command and control of the Army's fixed-facility medical, dental, and veterinary treatment facilities, providing preventive care, medical research and development and training institutions.

Structure and Subordinate Commands

MEDCOM is divided into Regional Medical Commands that oversee day-to-day operations in military treatment facilities, exercising command and control over the medical treatment facilities in their regions. There are currently five of these regional commands:

- Europe Regional Medical Command
- Southern Regional Medical Command
- Northern Regional Medical Command
- Pacific Regional Medical Command
- Western Regional Medical Command.

Additional subordinate commands of MEDCOM include:

- Army Medical Department Center & School (AMEDDC&S)
- U.S. Army Public Health Command (Provisional), (known as the U.S. Army Center for Health Promotion & Preventive Medicine prior to 1 October 2009 {USACHPPM or CHPPM})
- U.S. Army Medical Research and Materiel Command (USAMRMC)
- Warrior Transition Command (WTC)
- U.S. Army Dental Command (DENCOM)

Operations

In Garrison (Peacetime)

MEDCOM maintains day-to-day health care for soldiers, retired soldiers and the families of both. Despite the wide range of responsibilities involved in providing health care in traditional settings as well as on the battlefield, the Army Medical Department's quality of care compares very favorably with that of civilian health organizations, when measured by civilian standards. Many Army medical facilities report on their own quality-of-care standards on their individual Internet sites.

Deployments

When Army field hospitals deploy, most clinical professional and support personnel come from MEDCOM's fixed facilities. In addition to support of combat operations, deployments can be for humanitarian assistance, peacekeeping, and other stability and support operations. Under the Professional Officer Filler System (PROFIS), up to 26 percent of MEDCOM physicians and 43 percent of MEDCOM nurses are sent to field units during a full deployment. To replace PROFIS losses, Reserve units and Individual Mobilization Augmentees (non-unit reservists) are mobilized to work in medical treatment facilities. The department also provides trained medical specialists to the Army's combat medical units, which are assigned directly to combatant commanders.

Many Army Reserve and Army National Guard units deploy in support of the Army Medical Department. The Army depends heavily on its Reserve component for medical support—about 63 percent of the Army's medical forces are in the Reserve component.

Army Medical Department

The Army Medical Department of the U.S. Army (AMEDD) comprises the Army's six medical Special Branches (or "Corps") of officers and medical enlisted soldiers. It was established as the "Army Hospital" in July 1775 to coordinate the medical care required by the Continental Army during the Revolutionary War. The AMEDD is led by the Surgeon General of the U.S. Army, a lieutenant general.

The AMEDD is the U.S. Army's healthcare organization, not a U.S. Army command. The AMEDD is found in all three components of the Army: the Active Army, the U.S. Army Reserve, and the Army National Guard. Its headquarters are at Fort Sam Houston, San Antonio, Texas, which hosts the

AMEDD Center and School. Equal numbers of AMEDD senior leaders can be found in Washington D.C., divided between the Pentagon and the Walter Reed Army Medical Center (WRAMC).

The Academy of Health Sciences, under the Army Medical Department Center & School, provides training to the officers and enlisted soldiers of the AMEDD. As a result of BRAC 2005, enlisted medical training was transferred to the new Medical Education and Training Campus, consolidating most military enlisted medical training at Fort Sam Houston.[19]

Medical Special Branches

- Medical Corps (MC)
- Nurse Corps (AN)
- Dental Corps (DC)
- Veterinary Corps (VC)
- Medical Service Corps (MS)
- Medical Specialist Corps (AMSC)

United States Army Training and Doctrine Command

Established 1 July 1973, the United States Army Training and Doctrine Command (TRADOC) is an army command of the United States Army headquartered at Fort Monroe, Virginia. It is charged with overseeing training of Army forces, the development of operational doctrine, and the development and procurement of new weapons systems. TRADOC operates 33 schools and centers at 16 Army installations. TRADOC schools conduct 2,734 courses (81 directly in support of mobilization) and 373 language courses. The 2,734 courses include 503,164 seats for 434,424 soldiers; 34,675 other-service personnel; 7,824 international soldiers; and 26,241 civilians.[20]

TRADOC MissionThe official mission statement for TRADOC states:

> TRADOC develops the Army's Soldiers and Civilian leaders and designs, develops and integrates capabilities, concepts and

[19] U.S. Army Medical Department AMEDD Center and School Portal available on the Internet at: http://www.cs.amedd.army.mil/. Additional information specific to the Fort Sam Houston consolidation is available n the Internet at: http://www.aetc.af.mil/shared/media/document/AFD-071026-035.pdf
[20] TRADOC fact sheet available at: http://www.tradoc.army.mil/about.htm

> doctrine in order to build a campaign-capable, expeditionary Army in support of joint warfighting capability through Army Force Generation (ARFORGEN).[21]

TRADOC is the official command component that is responsible for training and developing the United States Army.

TRADOC History

TRADOC was established as a major U.S. Army command on 1 July 1973. The new command, along with the U.S. Army Forces Command (FORSCOM), was created from the Continental Army Command (CONARC) located at Fort Monroe, VA. That action was the major innovation in the Army's post-Vietnam reorganization, in the face of realization that CONARC's obligations and span of control were too broad for efficient focus. The new organization functionally realigned the major Army commands in the continental United States. CONARC, and Headquarters, U.S. Army Combat Developments Command (CDC), situated at Fort Belvoir, VA, were discontinued, with TRADOC and FORSCOM at Fort Belvoir assuming the realigned missions. TRADOC assumed the combat developments mission from CDC, took over the individual training mission formerly the responsibility of CONARC, and assumed command from CONARC of the major Army installations in the United States housing Army training center and Army branch schools. FORSCOM assumed CONARC's operational responsibility for the command and readiness of all divisions and corps in the continental U.S. and for the installations where they were based.

Joined under TRADOC, the major Army missions of individual training and combat developments each had its own lineage. The individual training responsibility had belonged, during World War II, to Headquarters Army Ground Forces (AGF). In 1946 numbered Army areas were established in the U.S. under AGF command. At that time, the AGF moved from Washington, D.C. to Fort Monroe, VA. In March 1948, the AGR was replaced at Fort Monroe with the new Office, Chief of Army Field Forces (OCAFF). OCAFF, however, did not command the training establishment. That function was exercised by Headquarters, Department of the Army through the numbered Armies to the corps, division, and Army Training Centers. In February 1955, HQ Continental Army Command (CONARC) replaced OCAFF, assuming its missions as well as the training missions from DA. In January, HQ CONARC was redesignated U.S. Continental Army Command. Combat developments

---

[21] TRADOC commander on ARFORGEN, and the US Army available at: http://www.tradoc.army.mil/about.htm

emerged as a formal Army mission in the early 1950s, and OCAFF assumed that role in 1952. In 1955, CONARC assumed the mission. In 1962, HQ U.S. Army Combat Development Command (CDC) was established to bring the combat developments function under one major Army command.[22]

TRADOC Priorities

1. Leader Development
2. Initial Military Training
3. Concepts and Capabilities Integration
4. Human Capital Enterprise
5. Army Training and Learning Concept
6. Doctrine

[22] TRADOC history available at: http://www.tradoc.army.mil/about.htm

Respiratory Diseases and Disorders

Subcourse MD0568

This page intentionally left blank.

U.S. ARMY MEDICAL DEPARTMENT CENTER AND SCHOOL
FORT SAM HOUSTON, TEXAS 78234-6100

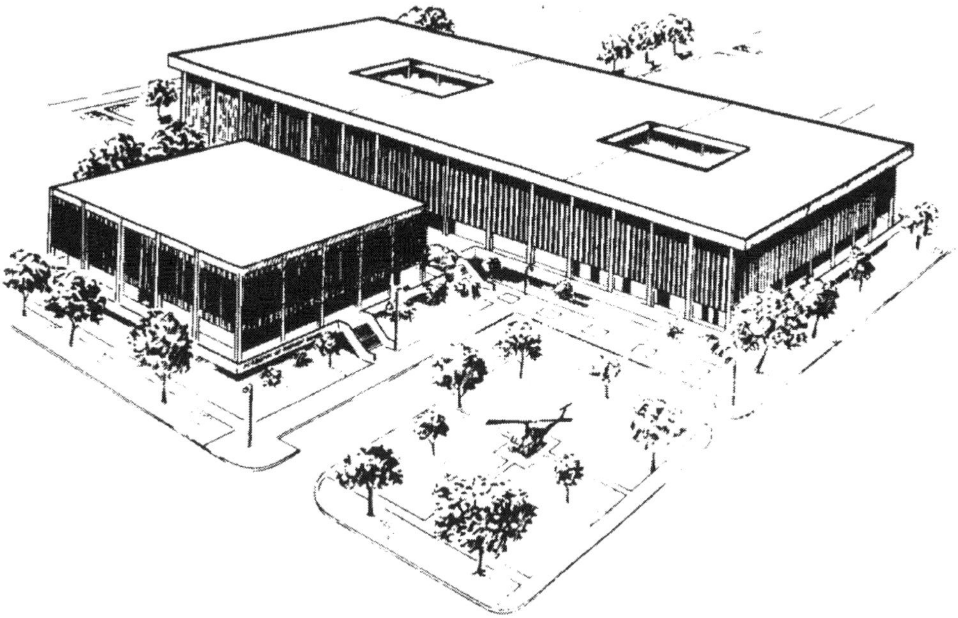

RESPIRATORY DISEASES AND DISORDERS

SUBCOURSE MD0568 EDITION 100

DEVELOPMENT

This subcourse is approved for resident and correspondence course instruction. It reflects the current thought of the Academy of Health Sciences and conforms to printed Department of the Army doctrine as closely as currently possible. Development and progress render such doctrine continuously subject to change.

The subject matter expert responsible for content accuracy of this edition was the NCOIC, Nursing Science Division, DSN 471-3086 or area code (210) 221-3086, M6 Branch, Academy of Health Sciences, ATTN: MCCS-HNP, Fort Sam Houston, Texas 78234-6100.

ADMINISTRATION

Students who desire credit hours for this correspondence subcourse must meet eligibility requirements and must enroll in the subcourse. Application for enrollment should be made at the Internet website: http://www.atrrs.army.mil. You can access the course catalog in the upper right corner. Enter School Code 555 for medical correspondence courses. Copy down the course number and title. To apply for enrollment, return to the main ATRRS screen and scroll down the right side for ATRRS Channels. Click on SELF DEVELOPMENT to open the application and then follow the on screen instructions.

For comments or questions regarding enrollment, student records, or examination shipments, contact the Nonresident Instruction Branch at DSN 471-5877, commercial (210) 221-5877, toll-free 1-800-344-2380; fax: 210-221-4012 or DSN 471-4012, e-mail accp@amedd.army.mil, or write to:

NONRESIDENT INSTRUCTION BRANCH
AMEDDC&S
ATTN: MCCS-HSN
2105 11TH STREET SUITE 4191
FORT SAM HOUSTON TX 78234-5064

CLARIFICATION OF TERMINOLOGY

When used in this publication, words such as "he," "him," "his," and "men" 'are intended to include both the masculine and feminine genders, unless specifically stated otherwise or when obvious in context.

TABLE OF CONTENTS

Lesson **Paragraphs**

INTRODUCTION

1 ANATOMY AND PHYSIOLOGY OF THE RESPIRATORY SYSTEM

Section I. Structure and Function of the Respiratory Organs.... 1-1--1-5
Section II. Accessory Structures of the Respiratory System...... 1-6--1-9
Section III. Physiology of Respiration 1-10--1-17
Exercises

2 PHYSICAL ASSESSMENT OF THE RESPIRATORY SYSTEM

Section I. General Approach to Physical Assessment 2-1--2-4
Section II. Steps of the Procedure.......... 2-5--2-8
Exercises

3 INFECTIOUS RESPIRATORY DISEASES

Section I. Upper Respiratory Diseases.................................... 3-1--3-5
Section II. Upper Respiratory Diseases with Systemic Effects 3-6--3-7
Section III. Lower Respiratory Diseases.................................... 3-8--3-10
Section IV. Other Causes of Pneumonia... 3-11--3-15
Exercises

4 CHRONIC OBSTRUCTIVE PULMONARY DISEASES

Section I. Asthma......................... 4-1--4-4
Section II. Chronic Bronchitis.............. 4-5--4-7
Section III. Emphysema.. 4-8--4-10
Exercises

5 RESPIRATORY DISORDERS

Section I. Hyperventilation Syndrome........ 5-1--5-3
Section II. Spontaneous Pneumothorax......... 5-4--5-7
Section III. Pulmonary Embolism... 5-8--5-12
Section IV. Inhaled Toxic Substances......... 5-13--5-17
Exercises

6 TUBERCULOSIS... 6-1--6-11
Exercises

CORRESPONDENCE COURSE OF
THE U.S. ARMY MEDICAL DEPARTMENT CENTER AND SCHOOL

SUBCOURSE MD0568

RESPIRATORY DISEASES AND DISORDERS

INTRODUCTION

The respiratory tract has defense mechanisms that prevent most microorganisms and foreign objects from entering the lungs of a healthy person. Sometimes these defense mechanisms cannot resist invasion, and infection occurs. The person's defenses may be weakened, damaged, or the invading agent may be too strong for the person's body to resist. As a Medical NCO, it is extremely important that you become aware of the characteristics and treatments for respiratory problems that you may encounter. With the awareness of respiratory diseases and their general characteristics, you may be alert for signs and symptoms of such diseases in the soldiers in your care.

Subcourse Components:

The subcourse instructional material consists of six lessons as follows:

Lesson 1, Anatomy and Physiology of the Respiratory System.
Lesson 2, Physical Assessment of the Respiratory System.
Lesson 3, Infectious Respiratory Diseases.
Lesson 4. Chronic Obstructive Pulmonary Diseases.
Lesson 5. Respiratory Disorders.
Lesson 6. Tuberculosis.

Here are some suggestions that may be helpful to you in completing this subcourse:

--Read and study each lesson carefully.

--Complete the subcourse lesson by lesson. After completing each lesson, work the exercises at the end of the lesson, marking your answers in this booklet.

--After completing each set of lesson exercises, compare your answers with those on the solution sheet that follows the exercises. If you have answered an exercise incorrectly, check the reference cited after the answer on the solution sheet to determine why your response was not the correct one.

Credit Awarded:

Upon successful completion of the examination for this subcourse, you will be awarded 12 credit hours.

To receive credit hours, you must be officially enrolled and complete an examination furnished by the Nonresident Instruction Branch at Fort Sam Houston, Texas.

You can enroll by going to the web site http://atrrs.army.mil and enrolling under "Self Development" (School Code 555).

A listing of correspondence courses and subcourses available through the Nonresident Instruction Section is found in Chapter 4 of DA Pamphlet 350-59, Army Correspondence Course Program Catalog. The DA PAM is available at the following website: http://www.usapa.army.mil/pdffiles/p350-59.pdf.

LESSON ASSIGNMENT

LESSON 1 Anatomy and Physiology of the Respiratory System.

TEXT ASSIGNMENT Paragraphs 1-1 through 1-17.

LESSON OBJECTIVES After completing this lesson, you should be able to:

1-1. Identify the structure and function of the respiratory organs.

1-2. Identify the accessory structures of the respiratory system.

1-3. Describe the physiology of respiration.

1-4. Describe factors in air capacity of the lungs.

SUGGESTION After completing the assignment, complete the exercises at the end of this lesson. These exercises will help you to achieve the lesson objectives.

LESSON 1

ANATOMY AND PHYSIOLOGY OF THE RESPIRATORY SYSTEM

Section I. STRUCTURE AND FUNCTION OF THE RESPIRATORY ORGANS

1-1. INTRODUCTION

a. **Respiration.** Respiration is the exchange of gases between the atmosphere and the cells of the body. It is a physiological process. There are two types of respiration: external respiration and internal respiration. External respiration is the exchange of gases between the air in the lungs and blood. Internal respiration is the exchange of gases between the blood and the individual cells of the body.

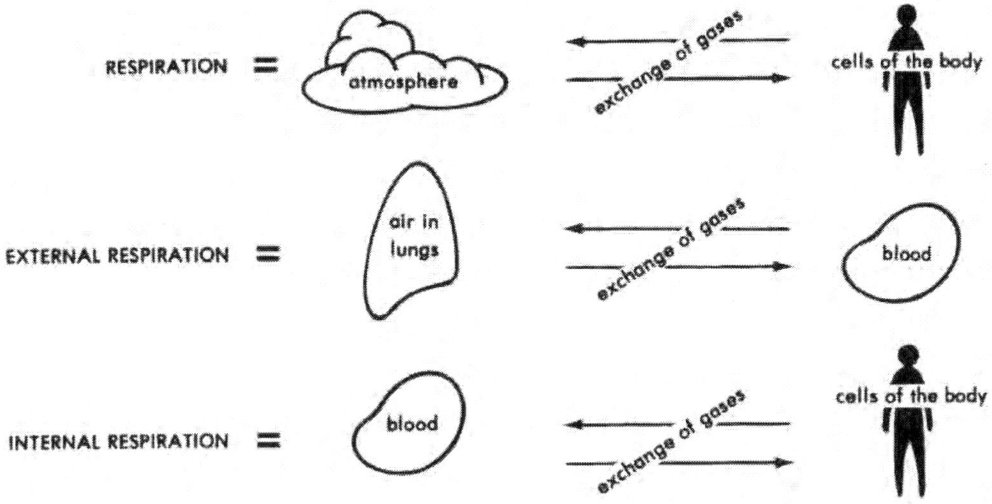

Figure 1-1. Respiration.

b. **Breathing.** Breathing is the process that moves air into and out of the lungs. It is a mechanical process. There are two types of breathing in humans: costal (thoracic) breathing and diaphragmatic (abdominal) breathing. In costal breathing, the major structure causing the movement of air is the rib cage. In diaphragmatic breathing, interaction between the diaphragm and the abdominal wall causes air to move into and out of the lungs.

```
COSTAL BREATHING =  air movement caused by rib cage

DIAPHRAGMATIC BREATHING =  diaphragm<--interaction-->abdominal wall
```

Figure 1-2. Breathing.

1-2. COMPONENTS AND SUBDIVISIONS OF THE HUMAN RESPIRATORY SYSTEM

See figure 1-3 for an illustration of the human respiratory system.

a. **Components.** The components of the human respiratory system consist of air passageways and two lungs. Air moves from the outside of the body into tiny sacs in the lungs called alveoli (pronounced al-VE-oh-lie).

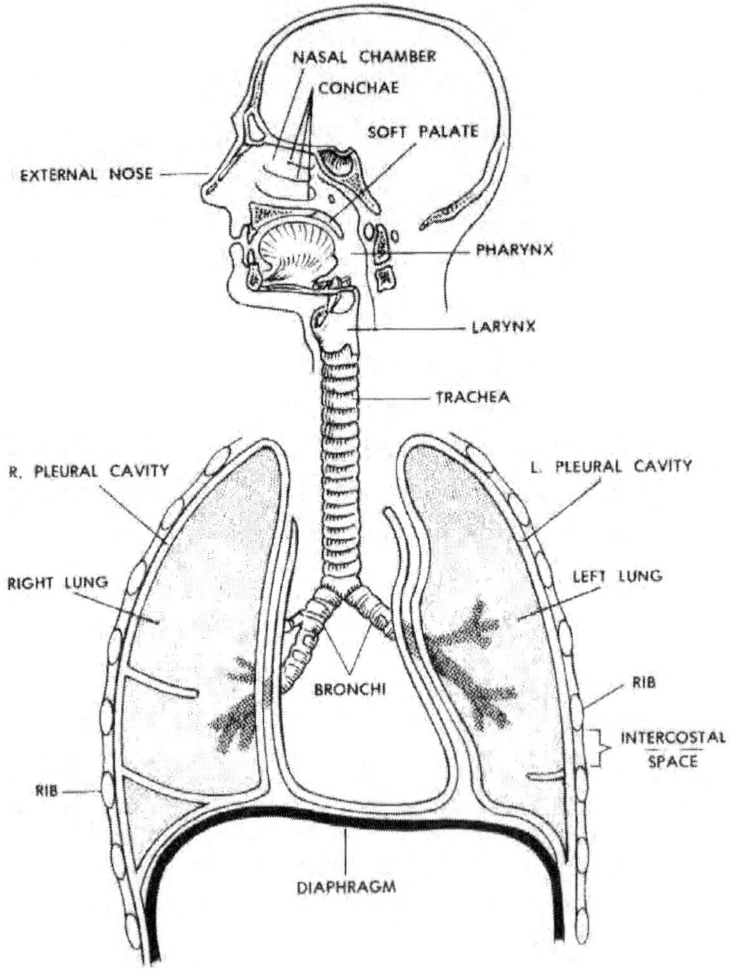

Figure 1-3. The human respiratory system.

b. **Main Subdivisions.** The main subdivisions of the respiratory system may be identified by their relationship to the voice box or larynx. Thus, the main subdivisions are as follows:

SUBDIVISION	FUNCTION
SUPRALARYNGEAL STRUCTURES (su-prah-lah-RIN-je-al)	Cleanse, warm, moisten, and test inflowing air.
LARYNX (voice-box) (LARE-inks)	Controls the volume of inflowing air; produces selected pitch (vibration frequency) in the moving column of air.
INFRALARYNGEAL STRUCTURES (in-frah-lah-RIN-je-al)	Distributes air to the alveoli of the lungs where actual respiration takes place.

1-3. SUPRALARYNGEAL STRUCTURES

See figure 1-4.

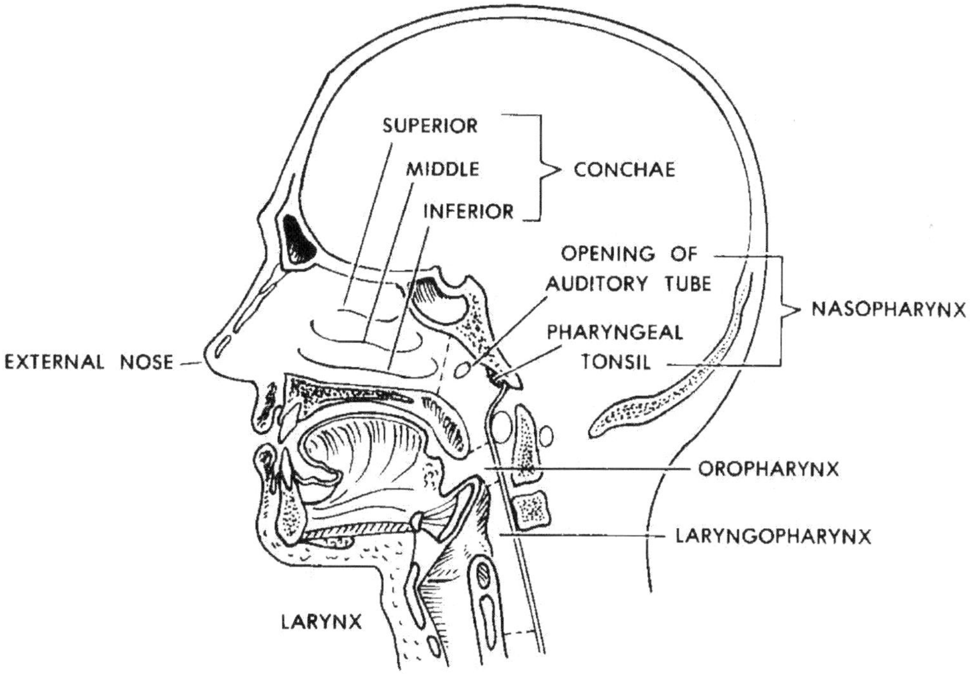

Figure 1-4. Supralaryngeal structures.

a. **Nose.** There is an external nose, the part projecting from the face, and an internal nose, the portion that is inside the skull.

(1) External portion of the nose. A supporting framework of bone and cartilage covered with skin and lined with mucous membrane makes up the external nose. Nasal bones form the bridge of the nose and hold it in a fixed position. The rest of the external nose is flexible because it has a framework of pliable cartilage. The midline divider of the external nose is called the nasal septum. Two openings called the nostrils or external nares are on the underside of the external nose. These nostrils lead to paired spaces (vestibules).

(2) Internal portion of the nose. Behind each vestibule of the external nose is a nasal chamber. The two chambers together form the internal nose. These chambers are separated by the nasal septum.

(a) Mucoperiosteum. The walls of the nasal chambers are lined with a thick mucous-type membrane known as the mucoperiosteum. This lining is moist and full of blood vessels. As air is inhaled and passes over this lining, several changes happen to the inhaled air. Blood in the lining's blood vessels warms the air. The air picks up moisture from the lining. Dust sticks to the mucous of the lining resulting in relatively dust-free air.

(b) Conchae. The lateral wall of each nasal chamber has three scroll-like extensions into the chamber, which help increase the surface area exposed to inflowing air. These scroll-like extensions are known as conchae.

CONCHA = sea shell pronounced KON-kah)

CONCHA (singular), Conchae (plural)

(c) Olfactory epithelium (membrane). The olfactory epithelium is a membrane that lines the upper nasal chambers. The olfactory receptors (nerve endings responsible for the sense of smell) are located in this membrane.

(d) Paranasal sinuses. Paranasal sinuses (figure 1-5) are air "cells" or cavities in the skull. They are connected with the nasal chambers and are lined with the same ciliated mucoperiosteum. These sinuses are extensions of the nasal chambers into the skull bones. For this reason, they are known as paranasal sinuses.

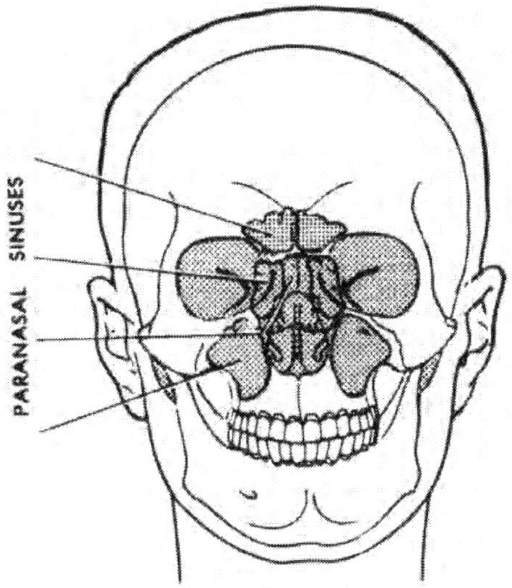

Figure 1-5. The nose.

b. **Pharynx.** The pharynx (FAIR-inks) is the common posterior space for the respiratory and digestive systems. It is about 13 cm or 5 inches long and is shaped a little like a funnel. It starts at the internal nares and extends partway down the neck. The wall of the pharynx is made up of skeletal muscles and lined with a mucous membrane.

(1) Function. The pharynx has two functions: it serves as a passageway for air and food, and it provides a resonating chamber (amplifying sounds) for speech sounds.

(2) Divisions. The pharynx can be divided into three parts: the nasopharynx, the oropharynx, and the laryngopharynx.

(a) Nasopharynx. The part of the pharynx specifically related to the respiratory system is the nasopharynx. It is located above the soft palate. The two posterior openings (nares or nostrils) of the nasal chambers lead into the single space of the nasopharynx. The auditory tubes (also called the eustachian tubes) open into the nasopharynx. The auditory tubes connect the nasopharynx with the middle ears to equalize the pressure between the outside and inside of the eardrum. The pharyngeal tonsils (adenoids) are located in the upper posterior wall of the nasopharynx. The soft palate, floor of the nasopharynx, is a trapdoor which closes off the upper respiratory passageways during swallowing.

(b) Oropharynx. This is the part of the pharynx which is closely related to the digestive system. It is located below the soft palate and above the upper edge of the epiglottis. (The epiglottis is the flap that prevents food from entering the larynx during swallowing.)

(c) Laryngopharynx. The part of the pharynx which is common to the respiratory and digestive systems is the laryngopharynx. It is the part of the pharynx below the edge of the epiglottis. The digestive and respiratory systems lead into this part from above and lead off from it below.

1-4. LARYNX

The larynx (figure 1-6), also called the voice box, connects the pharynx with the trachea. The larynx is located in the anterior region of the neck and has a box-like shape (see figure 1-3). The voice box of the male becomes larger and heavier during puberty causing the male's voice to get deeper. An adult male's voice box tends to be located lower in the neck than the female's voice box. The female's larynx remains higher and smaller causing the female's voice to be a higher pitch.

a. **Structure.** Nine pieces of cartilage support the larynx: three single pieces of cartilage and three paired pieces of cartilage. The three single pieces are the thyroid cartilage, epiglottic cartilage (epiglottis), and cricoid cartilage. The three paired pieces of cartilage are arytenoid cartilages, corniculate cartilages, and cuneiform cartilages.

(1) Thyroid cartilage. Sometimes called the Adam's apple, this cartilage is made up of two fused plates which form the anterior wall of the larynx. These plates cause the larynx to be triangular in shape. The thyroid cartilage is larger in males than in females.

(2) Epiglottic cartilage (epiglottis). This cartilage lies on top of the larynx and is shaped like a large leaf. The "stem" of the epiglottis is attached to the thyroid cartilage. The "leaf" of the epiglottis is unattached and moves up and down freely. During swallowing, the larynx moves up causing the free edge of the epiglottis to form a lid over the glottis, and the glottis is closed. The glottis is the hole between the vocal cords in the larynx. Air passes through the glottis into the main chamber of the larynx (below the cords) and then into the trachea. The covering over the glottis allows the larynx to be closed off. Liquids and foods then move into the esophagus and are kept out of the trachea. A cough reflex takes place in an effort to expel anything other than air that gets into the larynx.

(3) Cricoid (KRI-koyd) cartilage. This is a ring of cartilage that forms the interior wall of the larynx. It is attached to the first ring of the trachea.

(4) Arytenoid (ar-i-TE-noyd) cartilages (paired). The arytenoid cartilages are located at the superior border of the cricoid cartilage and are shaped like pyramids. These cartilages are attached to the vocal folds and pharyngeal muscles. The action of these cartilages causes the vocal cords to move.

(5) Corniculate (kor-NIK-yoo-lat) cartilages (paired). These cartilages are located at the apex of each arytenoid cartilage. They are shaped like a cone.

(6) Cuneiform (kyoo-NE-i-form) cartilages (paired). Cuneiform cartilages are shaped like rods. These cartilages connect the epiglottis to the arytenoid cartilages.

b. **Voice Cords.** The mucous membrane of the larynx contains two pairs of folds: the superior folds (false vocal cords) and the inferior folds (true vocal cords).

(1) Superior folds (false vocal cords). If these folds are brought together, they function in holding the breath against pressure in the thoracic cavity. Humans hold their breath when they push against something heavy or pick up a heavy object.

(2) Inferior folds (true vocal cords). The movement of air across these vocal cords produces sounds. Tension on the vocal cords controls pitch. Men usually have thicker and longer vocal folds. This causes the vocal folds to vibrate more slowly giving males a lower range of pitch than females.

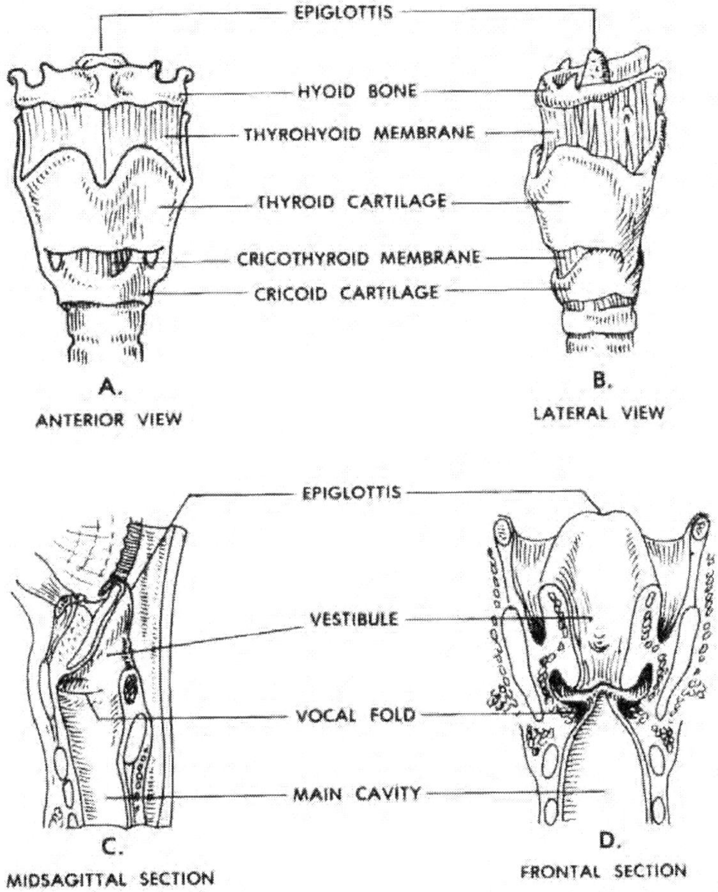

Figure 1-6. The larynx.

1-5. INFRALARYNGEAL STRUCTURES

a. **Trachea and Bronchi.** The respiratory tree (figure 1-7) is the set of tubular structures that carry air from the larynx to the alveoli of the lungs. If you were to turn figure 1-7 UPSIDE DOWN, the trachea would become the trunk of the tree, and the bronchi would be the branches. (NOTE: Figure 1-7 is right side up.) These tubular parts are held open by rings of cartilage. The lining is ciliated to remove mucus and other materials that get into the passageway.

b. **Alveoli.** The alveoli (alveolus, singular) are tiny round (balloon-like) sacs that are connected to larger tubes of the lungs by tiny tubes known as alveolar ducts and bronchioles. The alveoli are so small that there are billions in adult lungs. This very small size produces a maximum surface area through which external respiration takes place. External respiration is the actual exchange of gases between the air in the alveolar spaces and the adjacent blood capillaries through their walls. The inner surfaces of the alveoli must be kept wet in order for this transfer of gases to be possible.

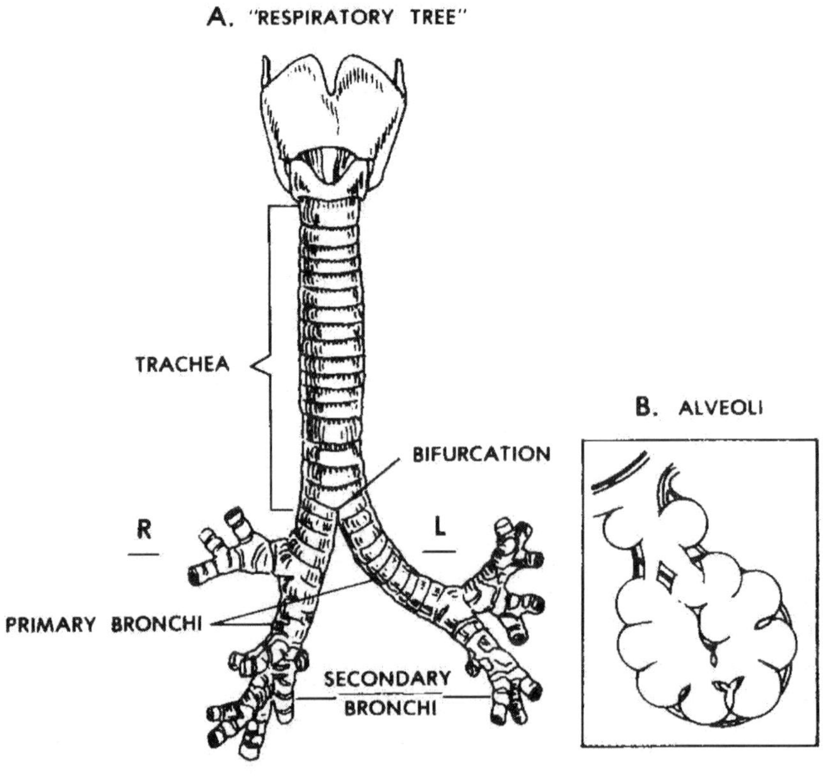

Figure 1-7. Infralaryngeal structures ("respiratory tree").

c. **Lungs.** A lung is an individual organ composed of tubular structures and alveoli bound together by porous, spongy, elastic type, fibrous connective tissue. In humans, there are two lungs: the right lung and the left lung. Each lung is supplied by a primary or mainstem bronchus leading off the trachea.

(1) Structure. The right lung is larger in volume and shorter than the left lung. The left lung must leave room for the heart. The right lung is divided into three pulmonary lobes (upper, middle and lower) and 10 bronchopulmonary segments (2 + 3 + 5). The left lung is smaller and narrower than the right lung and is divided into two pulmonary lobes (upper and lower) and eight bronchopulmonary segments (4 + 4). A pulmonary lobe is a major subdivision of a lung marked by fissures (deep folds). Each lobe is further partitioned into bronchopulmonary segments. Each lobe is supplied by a secondary or lobar bronchus. Each segment is supplied by a tertiary or segmental bronchus, a branch of the lobar bronchus.

(2) Lung lobules. Each bronchopulmonary segment of the lung is divided into many small compartments called lobules. See figure 1-8. Elastic connective tissue is wrapped around each lobule. Each lobule has a lymphatic vessel, an arteriole, a venule, and a branch from a terminal bronchioles. Terminal bronchioles further subdivide into tiny branches called respiratory bronchioles. Respiratory bronchioles subdivide into several (2 to 11) alveolar ducts. Many alveoli and alveolar sacs surround the alveolar duct.

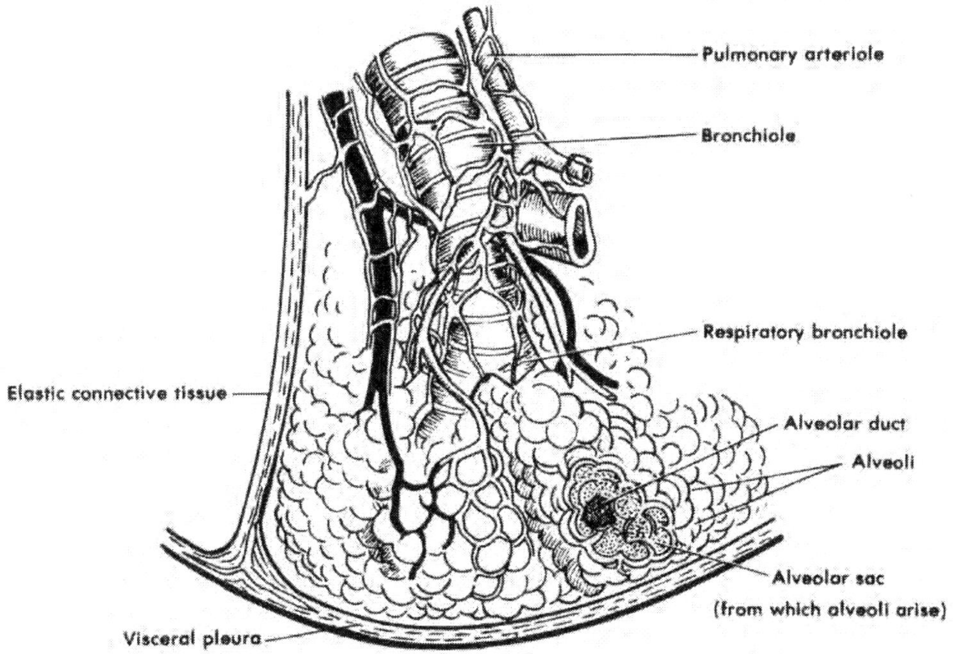

Figure 1-8. Diagram of a lung lobule.

Section II. ACCESSORY STRUCTURES OF THE RESPIRATORY SYSTEM

NOTE: All of the structures in this section play a part in the functioning of the respiratory system.

1-6. DIAPHRAGM

The diaphragm, the chief muscle of respiration, is a thin, but strong, dome-shaped muscular membrane. It separates the abdominal and thoracic cavities. The diaphragm is attached to the inferior margin of the rib cage and to the bodies of the lumbar vertebrae behind. As a muscular membrane, it domes upward into the thoracic cavity. Upon contraction, the fibers of the diaphragm shorten and pull downward. This downward motion produces a piston-like pressure on the contents of the abdominopelvic cavity.

1-7. INTERCOSTAL MUSCLES

a. The intercostal spaces are filled by two layers of intercostal muscles. The intercostal muscles extend from the vertebrae behind to the sternum in front. A strengthening "plywood effect" is created by the arrangement of the two layers at a right angle to each other. These muscles help maintain the "solid-wall" condition of the thorax. For this reason, a pressure gradient can be maintained between the inside and outside of the thorax.

b. The intercostal muscles play a part in the mechanics of breathing. Quiet breathing takes place due to the alternate contraction and relaxation of the diaphragm and the internal intercostal muscles. As an individual breathes in, the diaphragm contracts and, at the same time, the external intercostal muscles contract causing the ribs to be pulled upward and the sternum to be pushed forward. This increases the anterior-posterior diameter of the thoracic cavity. (The volume of the chest cavity increases.) When the individual breathes out, the external intercostal muscles relax, the ribs move downward, and, as the diaphragm relaxes, the thoracic cage moves upward. These movements decrease the vertical and anterior-posterior diameters of the thoracic cavity. The thoracic cavity (smaller in volume) returns to its resting size.

1-8. THORAX

The thorax is the chest. The thorax is the portion of the trunk consisting of the sternum, the costal cartilages, the ribs, and the bodies of the thoracic vertebrae. Located above the diaphragm, the thoracic cage is roughly cone-shaped, the narrow portion being superior and the broad portion inferior. It is flattened from front to back. The thoracic cage is open to the outside by way of the neck and head. This bony cage encloses and protects the lungs and other structures of the chest cavity. The thorax also provides support for the bones of the shoulder girdle and upper extremities. Since the wall of the thorax is reinforced by special muscles, bones, and cartilages, we can consider the thorax to be a "solid-walled container."

1-9. PLEURA

Surrounding each lung individually is a serous cavity called the pleural cavity (figure 1-9). The minute quantity of serous fluid in the cavity serves as a lubricant. This serves to minimize friction for the expansion and contraction of the lungs during breathing.

a. Each lung is covered with a serous membrane called the visceral pleura. The outer wall of the pleural cavity is lined with another serous membrane known as the parietal pleura. Areas of the parietal pleura are variously named according to their location. The mediastinal pleura form the lateral wall of the mediastinum. The diaphragmatic pleura cover the superior surface of the diaphragm. The costal pleura line the inner surface of the rib cage. The cupolar pleura form a dome-like extension into the root of the neck. It contains the apex of the lung.

b. When each lung is in its smaller volume, its corresponding diaphragmatic pleura lies close to the lower costal pleura. The slit-like cavity between them is called the costophrenic sinus. Fluids of each pleural cavity tend to collect in this sinus since it is the lowest area for each. When the diaphragm contracts and flattens out, each costophrenic sinus opens up, and the inferior portion of the expanding lung occupies this space.

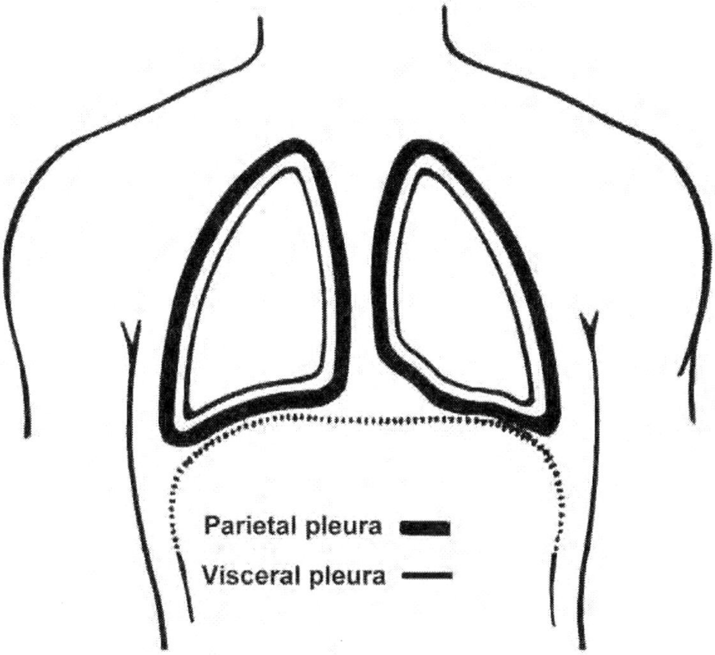

Figure 1-9. Lungs, visceral, and parietal pleura.

Section III. PHYSIOLOGY OF RESPIRATION

1-10. INTRODUCTION

a. Boyle's law tells us that as the volume (V) of a gas-filled container increases, the pressure (P) inside decreases; as the volume (V) of a closed container decreases, the pressure (P) inside increases. When the connected spaces of air have different pressures, the air moves from the space with greater pressure to the one with lesser pressure.

b. In regard to breathing, we can consider the air pressure around the human body to be constant. The pressure inside the lungs may be greater or less than the pressure outside the body. Thus, a greater internal pressure causes air to flow out; a greater external pressure causes air to flow in.

c. We can compare the human trunk to a hollow cylinder. This cylinder is divided into upper and lower cavities by the diaphragm. The upper is the thoracic cavity and is essentially gas-filled. The lower is the abdominopelvic cavity and is essentially water-filled.

1-11. COSTAL (THORACIC) BREATHING

a. **Inhalation.** Muscles attached to the thoracic cage raise the rib cage. A typical rib might be compared to a bucket handle, attached at one end to the sternum (breastbone) and at the other end to the vertebral column. The "bucket handle" is lifted by the overall movement upward and outward of the rib cage. These movements increase the thoracic diameters from right to left and from front to back. Thus, the intrathoracic volume increases. Recalling Boyle's law, the increase in volume leads to a decrease in pressure. The air pressure outside the body then forces air into the lungs and inflates them.

b. **Exhalation.** The rib cage movements and pressure relationships are reversed for exhalation. Thus, intrathoracic volume decreases. The intrathoracic pressure increases and forces air outside the body.

1-12. DIAPHRAGMATIC (ABDOMINAL) BREATHING

a. **Inhalation.** As the diaphragm contracts, the dome flattens, and the diaphragm descends. This increases the depth (vertical diameter) of the thoracic cavity thus increasing the cavity's volume. At the same time, air pressure in the thoracic cavity decreases. Now, air pressure outside the body is greater, a condition which forces air into the lungs.

b. **Exhalation.** As the diaphragm relaxes, the elastic abdominal wall forces the diaphragm back up by pushing the watery tissues of the abdomen against the underside of the relaxed diaphragm. The dome extends upward. Air is forced out of the lungs.

1-13. CARBON DIOXIDE TRANSPORT AND ELIMINATION

a. **The Reason for Breathing.** Humans breath to supply oxygen to the cells of the body and to remove the waste product, carbon dioxide (CO_2). About one-fifth of the air around us is oxygen. In the process of breathing, or respiration, the body brings air into the lungs. In the lungs, some of the oxygen moves into the bloodstream. A waste gas, carbon dioxide, moves from the blood into the air in the lungs where it is breathed out. The name of this process is the exchange of gases.

b. **The Exchange of Gases.** The actual exchange of oxygen and carbon dioxide takes place in tiny air sacs, the alveoli. The alveoli are in direct contact with capillaries that carry blood. The alveoli walls and the capillary walls are moist and very thin--much thinner than tissue paper. Oxygen molecules seep from the alveoli through the membranes (thin walls) into the blood of the capillaries. Hemoglobin picks up oxygen in the red blood cells. At the same time, blood plasma gives up carbon dioxide to the air in the alveoli. Figure 1-10 illustrates this exchange.

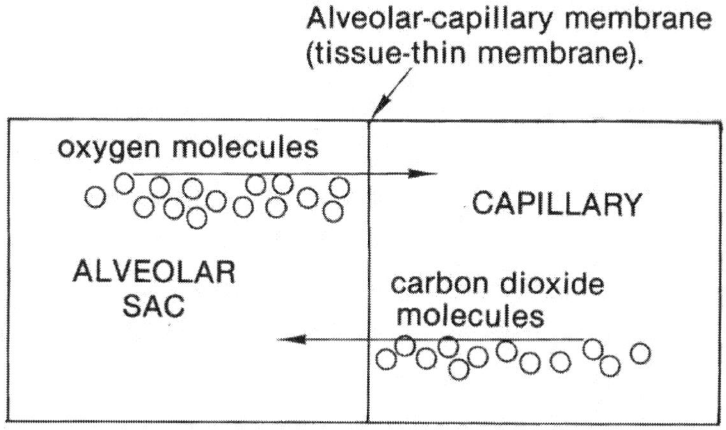

Figure 1-10. Exchange of gases.

1-14. REGULATION OF RESPIRATION

The basic rhythm is set and coordinated by the respiratory center; however, the rhythm can be modified in response to the demands of the body by the nerve (neural) center.

RESPIRATORY CENTER =	neurons (any of the conducting cells of the nervous system) in the reticular formation of the brain stem that regulate the rate of respiration.
VENTILATION =	the volume of air exchanged in one minute.

a. **Brain Influences** (Cortical Influences). The brain can send a message to the respiratory center allowing humans to voluntarily control breathing and even stop breathing for a short time. The fact that we can voluntarily stop breathing is a protection because in this way we can keep water or irritating gases from entering our lungs. However, when CO_2 builds up to a certain level in our blood, impulses are sent to the inspiratory muscles, causing us to breathe whether we want to or not. It is not possible to kill yourself by holding your breath.

b. **Medullary Rhythmicity Area.** This area controls the basic rhythm of respiration. The respiratory center in the medulla (an inner layer of an organ) adjusts the alveolar ventilation almost exactly to the demands of the body. The result is that there is hardly any change of oxygen and carbon dioxide in arterial blood. The respiratory center of the medulla or its immediate vicinity is the primary site of action of carbon dioxide and hydrogen ions. Reduced oxygen concentrations in the blood stimulate chemoreceptors (a receptor sensitive to chemical changes in the blood stream). Impulses are transmitted to the respiratory center to increase ventilation (the volume of air exchanged in one minute) when these receptors are stimulated. Normally, the increase in ventilation prevents a rise in carbon dioxide to the point that the respiratory center would be stimulated.

1-15. FACTORS THAT CAN DECREASE OXYGEN TRANSPORT TO TISSUES

a. **Decreased Levels of Hb.** Hb is reduced hemoglobin (hemoglobin that has not combined with oxygen). Since oxygen does not dissolve well in water, very little oxygen can be carried by water through the body. Hb (hemoglobin) combines with oxygen and carries about 97 percent of the needed oxygen to various parts of the body. If there is less Hb in the body to combine with and carry oxygen around, there will necessarily be less oxygen transported to tissues of the body.

b. **Cardiac Failure.** The cardiovascular system transports gases in the blood between the lungs and the cells. The heart pumps blood carrying oxygen through the body. The cells of the body cannot survive long if they are starved for blood carrying oxygen. If oxygen is withheld from the cells of the brain for 5 to 6 minutes, a person can suffer severe and permanent brain injury or death.

c. **Decreased Rate of Respiration.** In order for a human to survive, there must be a continuous supply of oxygen to the blood as well as a continuous removal of carbon dioxide from the body. Respiration, the inhaling of oxygen and expelling of carbon dioxide, takes care of the oxygen and carbon dioxide levels in the body. If the respiration rate is lowered, an individual may have enough oxygen but too much carbon dioxide in the body.

d. **Disease Processes of Lungs or Component Parts.**

(1) Lung cancer. People inhale many irritating substances as a part of ordinary breathing. Inhaled smoke and almost all pollutants have an irritating effect on the bronchial tubes and lungs. These pollutants act as stresses or irritating stimuli. A common lung cancer, bronchogenic carcinoma, starts in the walls of the bronchi and is caused by stress and irritation.

(2) Nasal polyps. These polyps, protruding growths of mucous membrane hanging down from the posterior wall of the nasal septum, are bluish-white tumors. As they become larger, they may fill the nasopharynx making breathing through the nose difficult. A doctor can remove these polyps easily.

(3) Bronchial asthma. Usually, bronchial asthma is caused by an allergy to edible or air-borne substances--for example, wheat or dust. Muscles in the walls of the small bronchi and bronchioles go into spasms caused by the allergy. Also, the smaller bronchi and bronchioles may be clogged with excessive amounts of mucous making breathing difficult.

(4) Bronchitis. Bronchitis is inflammation of the bronchi. The most important cause of chronic bronchitis is cigarette smoking. (Chronic bronchitis is bronchitis that lasts for at least three months of the year for two successive years.)

(5) Emphysema. In this disease, the alveolar walls lose their elasticity and remain filled with air during expiration. The word "emphysema" means "blown up" or "full of air." A person with emphysema must actively work to exhale. Also, as a result of damage to the alveolar-capillary membrane, the respiration rate slows down. Removing the irritating stimuli-- air pollution, occupational exposure to dust, cigarette smoking--can slow down the progressive deterioration.

(6) Pneumonia. Pneumonia is an acute infection or inflammation of the alveoli. The amount of air space in the lungs is reduced because the alveolar sacs fill up with fluid and dead white cells. A bacteria called pneumococcus bacterium is the most common cause of this disease, but other bacteria or a fungus may also cause pneumonia. Several viruses may cause viral pneumonia.

(7) Tuberculosis. Tuberculosis is caused by a bacteria-- Mycobacterium tuberculosis--which destroys parts of the lung tissue. Tuberculosis bacteria are spread by inhaling, can live through some disinfectants, but are killed by sunlight. This disease is sometimes associated with crowded, poorly lit housing. A person with tuberculosis must have rest, sunlight, and good diet.

(8) Coryza (common cold) and Influenza (flu). Common colds are caused by viruses and typical symptoms include sneezing, excessive nasal secretion, and congestion. (A fever is not usually one of the symptoms.) A virus also causes influenza (flu) with accompanying symptoms of chills, fever (usually higher than 101ºF), headache, and muscular aches. As the fever subsides, cold-like symptoms appear.

1-16. RESPIRATORY CYCLE

a. A respiratory cycle (figure 1-11) consists of one inspiration, one rest period, and one expiration--in that order.

Inspiration	(intake of air or inhaling)
Rest period	(between inspiration and expiration)
+ Expiration	(exhaling)
RESPIRATION CYCLE	(12 to 20 respiration cycles per minute)

Figure 1-11. Respiratory cycle.

b. Air is made up of several gases, the most important being oxygen. Carbon dioxide and nitrogen are also present along with some other gases in small amounts. The air we breathe in is not the same as the air we breathe out. Look at the gases in the air in figure 1-12 below.

Air breathed in	(inhaled)	Air breathed out (exhaled)
Nitrogen	79.02%	79.2%
Oxygen	20.94%	16.3%
Carbon Dioxide	0.04%	4.5%

Figure 1-12. Gases in the air.

c. You can see that air breathed out has less oxygen than air breathed in. The body has used some of the oxygen. Air breathed out has more carbon dioxide than air breathed in. The body is expelling carbon dioxide that has been formed as body cells work and use up oxygen.

1-17. AIR CAPACITY OF THE LUNGS

The amount of air in the lung of a man of average size who is resting is about 3 liters. When the man breathes in (inspiration or inhalation), he pulls in about 500 milliliters of air. When he deliberately breathes in (forced maximum inspiration), the amount of air in the lung rises to about 6 liters. When the same man forces the maximum amount of air out of the lung, the volume of air is down to about 1 liter. Here are important facts about volume of air and the lungs:

NOTE: 1 milliliter (ml) = 1 cubic centimeter (cc).

a. The total capacity of the lungs is about 6,000cc (maximum).

b. Tidal air volume is the amount of air inhaled or exhaled with each breath, whether the body is at rest or engaged in an activity. For the average adult male who is resting, the tidal volume is about 500cc of air.

c. Reserve air is air in the lungs that can be exhaled after normal exhalation. The amount of this air is about 1,500cc.

d. Residual air is air that is in the lungs after normal, forceful expiration (about 1,200cc).

e. Vital capacity (usually 4,800cc) is the volume of air that can be expelled after full inspiration.

Continue with Exercises

EXERCISES, LESSON 1

INSTRUCTIONS: Answer these exercises by writing the answer in the space provided. After you have answered all the exercises, turn to "Solutions to Exercises" at the end of the lesson and check your answers.

1. The exchange of gases between the atmosphere and the cells of the body is

   ____.

2. The exchange of gases between the air in the lungs and the blood is

   ____..

3. The exchange of gases between the blood and individual cells of the body is

   ____.

4. The process that moves air into and out of the lungs is a mechanical process

   called ____.

5. In __________________________ breathing, air movement is caused by the rib

   cage; in _____________________________ breathing, movement between the abdominal wall and the diaphragm cause air movement in and out of the lungs.

6. The main subdivisions of the respiratory system are the supralaryngeal

   structures, the ________________ and the __________________ structures.

7. The paranasal sinuses are ____.

8. The olfactory epithelium, a membrane lining the ___________________, houses

   the nerve endings responsible for the _____________________________.

9. The ________________________ is the portion of the nose inside the skull.

10. The three parts of the pharynx are the ________________________________,

______________________, and the ____________________________.

11. The _________________________ cartilage is a ring of cartilage forming the interior wall of the larynx.

12. The ______________________________ cartilage is larger in males than females and causes the larynx to be triangular shaped.

13. The trachea and the bronchi are tubular structures which carry air from the larynx

to _________________________________.

14. A lung is an individual organ composed of ___________________structures and

__________________ bound together by porous, spongy, elastic-type, fibrous connective tissue.

15. ____________________________is a membrane enfolding lungs and lining the walls of the chest cavity.

16. Humans can voluntarily control breathing and even stop breathing for a short

time because the brain sends a message to the _____________________.

17. Three factors which could decrease oxygen transportation to body tissues are

decreased levels of Hb, c___________f_____________ and

d_______________r_______________of r___________________.

18. Air breathed out has more carbon dioxide than air breathed in because

____________________________________.

19. The total capacity of the lungs is about _______________________ cc.

20. Vital capacity of the lungs (usually about 4,800 cc) is __________________________

____

21. The inner surfaces of the alveoli must be kept wet to ______________________

__________________________.

22. The chief muscle of respiration is the ____________________________________.

Check Your Answers on Next Page

SOLUTIONS TO EXERCISES, LESSON 1

1. Respiration. (para 1-1a)

2. External respiration. (para 1-1a)

3. Internal respiration. (para 1-1a)

4. Breathing. (para 1-1b)

5. Costal; diaphragmatic. (para 1-1b)

6. Larynx; infralaryngeal. (para 1-2b(1) through (3))

7. Air cells or cavities in the skull. (para 1-3a(2)(d))

8. Upper nasal chambers; sense of smell. (para 1-3a(2)(c))

9. Internal nose. (para 1-3a(2))

10. Nasopharynx, oropharynx, laryngopharynx. (para 1-3b(2))

11. Cricoid. (para 1-4a(3))

12. Thyroid. (para 1-4a(1))

13. The alveoli of the lungs. (para 1-5a)

14. Tubular; alveoli. (para 1-5c)

15. Pleura. (para 1-9)

16. Respiratory center. (para 1-14a)

17. Cardiac failure; decreased rate of respiration. (para 1-15a, b, c)

18. The body is expelling carbon dioxide that has been formed as the body cells work and use up oxygen. (para 1-16c)

19. 6,000. (para 1-17a)

20. The volume of air that can be expelled after a full inspiration. (para 1-17e)

21. Make the transfer of gases possible. (para 1-5b)
22. Diaphragm. (para 1-6)

End of Lesson 1

LESSON ASSIGNMENT

LESSON 2 Physical Assessment of the Respiratory System.

LESSON ASSIGNMENT Paragraphs 2-1 through 2-8.

LESSON OBJECTIVES After completing this lesson, you should be able to:

2-1. Perform the preliminary steps in physical assessment of the respiratory system.

2-2. Perform these examination techniques: inspection, palpation, percussion, auscultation.

SUGGESTION After completing the assignment, complete the exercises at the end of this lesson. These exercises will help you to achieve the lesson objectives.

LESSON 2

PHYSICAL ASSESSMENT OF THE RESPIRATORY SYSTEM

Section I. GENERAL APPROACH TO PHYSICAL ASSESSMENT

2-1. PATIENT'S HISTORY

The patient's history, obtained by interviewing him, is the patient's view of his health problems, general health condition, past medical history, family health history, and profile of his personal and social life and well-being. Additionally, the patient's history will show information the patient knows about his health, what is important in terms of health care, and what he expects from the health care being asked for. Since the interviewer is getting the information from the patient rather than observing him directly, the patient history information is subjective information. Be sure to record this information immediately and in an organized manner.

2-2. CONDITIONS

The patient should be undressed to the waist. Be sure the examination is conducted in a room with good light.

2-3. PROCEDURE

a. Working from the top of the patient's body down, perform the examination systematically from the head to the foot. In this way, you will be thorough and not miss anything.

b. Compare the findings on one side of the body with the findings on the other side of the body. In many instances, the body is bilaterally symmetrical; that is, the left side of the body has many of the same parts as the right side of the body. The parts are arranged as if the right side had been turned over.

c. Throughout the examination, try to visualize the structure of the body parts underneath the tissues. In each region of the body, consider the function of the body parts and be alert for any abnormalities.

d. Examine the patient's posterior thorax and lungs while he is in the sitting position. The patient's arms should be folded across his chest so that the scapulae (the shoulder blades) are partly out of the way. Then ask the patient to lie down while you examine his anterior thorax and lungs.

2-4. FUNCTIONS OF THE PHYSICAL ASSESSMENT

There are four functions (or parts) of the physical assessment: inspection, palpation, percussion, and auscultation. When you are doing a physical assessment, perform these functions in the order just given. The definition of each function is given in figure 2-1.

INSPECTION	=	Looking at the patient and observing the patient's behavior and body.
PALPATION	=	Touching the patient's body and noting what the various structures and parts of the body feel like.
PERCUSSION	=	Striking parts of the patient's body with short, sharp blows, and listening to the sounds of the body parts underneath the tissues.
AUSCULTATION	=	Using the stethoscope to listen to sounds in the body.

Figure 2-1. Techniques of examination/assessment.

Section II. STEPS OF THE PROCEDURE

2-5. INSPECTION

Inspection, the most important of the examination techniques, begins with the first moment you see the patient. Begin each portion of the examination by looking at the part of the body you are examining.

a. **The Patient**. The patient should be calm, relaxed, and not unduly apprehensive.

b. **Breathing**. Observe the patient for these aspects of breathing:

(1) Respiratory rate. The respiratory rate should be between 12 and 20 breaths per minute with even and easy movements of the respiratory muscles and chest expansion.

(2) Rhythm. Note the rhythm of the patient's breathing.

(3) Breathing. Note whether or not it is an effort for the patient to breath.

c. **Skin**. Look at the color of the patient's skin and check for bruises and/or lacerations.

d. **Chest**. Observe the shape of the patient's chest. The chest should be bilaterally symmetrical.

e. **Respirations**. Respirations should be the result of movement of the diaphragm.

2-6. PALPATION

Palpation is touching the part of the patient's body you have just inspected and becoming sensitive to what that body part feels like. It is possible to feel an abnormal from a normal body part.

a. **Four Uses for Palpation of the Chest**.

(1) Identify areas of tenderness. Any area where the patient has reported pain or where there are lesions (a hurt, injury, wound) should be palpated.

(2) Assess observed abnormalities. If you have seen masses or sinus tracts (blind, inflammatory, tube-like structures opening into the skin), palpate the area to evaluate the problem further.

(3) Further assess the respiratory excursion. Determine the range of respiratory movement (how far the chest expands when he inhales and how far the chest contracts when he exhales). You can also feel symmetry of respiratory movement (whether or not the body parts feel the same on both sides during a respiration).

REMEMBER: 1 RESPIRATION = 1 INHALATION + 1 EXHALATION

(4) Elicit tactile fremitus. When a person speaks, vibrations that can be felt are transmitted through the bronchopulmonary system to the chest wall. These vibrations can best be felt when a person says the words "ninety-nine" or "one-one-one." Ask the person to speak louder or lower his head if you cannot feel the vibrations.

b. **Finger Placement**. Place your finger pads on the skin surface over the area you are palpating. Do not move your fingers over the skin surface during palpation. Palpation should reveal a chest free from pain, tenderness, lesions, and masses. The wall should be firm with no indication of rib fractures or abscesses. The trachea will be midline; a deviated trachea is abnormal. Palpation of the respiratory excursion (respiration at rest position) should reveal an even, symmetrical movement of the chest.

c. **Assessment of Respiratory Excursion**.

(1) Posterior (figure 2-2).

(a) Place your thumbs about the level of and parallel to the 10th rib, your hands grasping the lateral rib cage.

(b) As you position your hands, slide them medially in order to raise loose skin folds between your thumbs and the patient's spine.

(c) Feel for range of symmetry of respiratory movement.

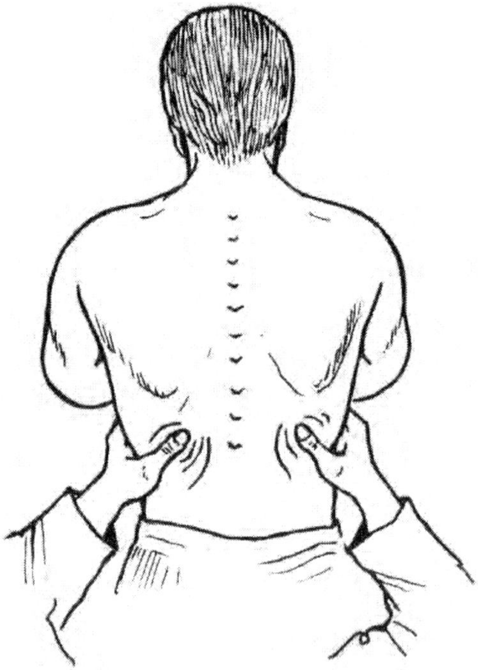

Figure 2-2. Posterior palpation.

(2) Anterior (figure 2-3).

(a) Place your thumbs along each costal margin with your hands along the lateral rib cage.

(b) As you position your hands, slide them medially a bit to raise a loose skin fold between the thumbs.

(c) Ask the patient to inhale deeply.

(d) Watch for your thumbs to separate as the thorax expands.

(e) Feel for the range and symmetry of respiratory movement.

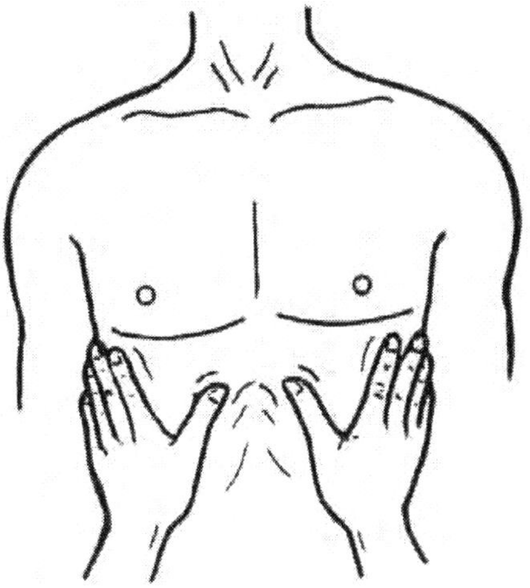

Figure 2-3. Anterior palpation.

d. **Palpate the Chest for Tactile Fremitus** (figure 2-4). Fremitus refers to the palpable vibrations transmitted through the lungs to the chest wall when the patient speaks. Have the patient say "ninety-nine" or "one-one-one" and you will feel vibrations. Vibrations are more difficult to feel over bone. NOTE: Patients with a heavy layer of fat may need to speak more loudly for you to feel the vibrations.

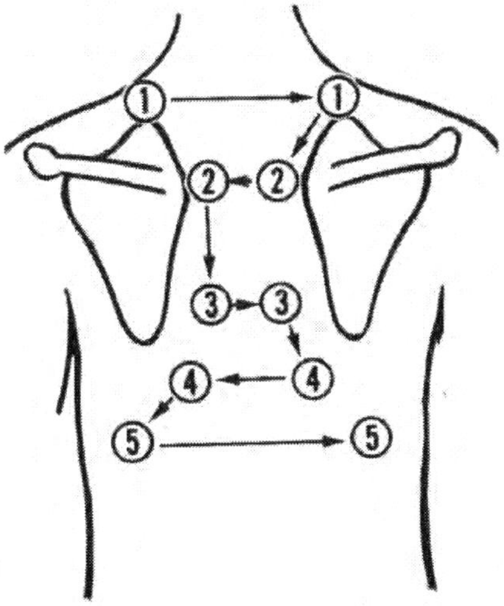

Figure 2-4. Sequence of tactile fremitus examination.

e. **Follow this Procedure to Palpate Properly.**

(1) Use the ball of the hand (the palm of the hand at the base of the fingers), palpate and compare like areas of the lungs. To be more accurate, use only one hand rather than both hands. Do not let your fingers touch the patient's chest.

(2) Have the patient repeat a sound that will make full and rich sounds such as "ninety-nine" or "one-one-one." Symmetrically move your hand over the patient's chest.

(3) You should feel vibrations of equal intensity on either side of the patient's chest.

(4) Normally, you will feel fremitus on the upper chest, close to the bronchi.

(5) Also, normally, you should feel little or no fremitus in the lower chest.

(6) Compare like (symmetrical) areas of the lungs.

f. **Diaphragm Level** (figure 2-5). The level of the diaphragm can be estimated roughly by noting where fremitus stops upon the downward palpation of the chest. It is normal to find that the right side of the diaphragm is slightly higher than the left side.

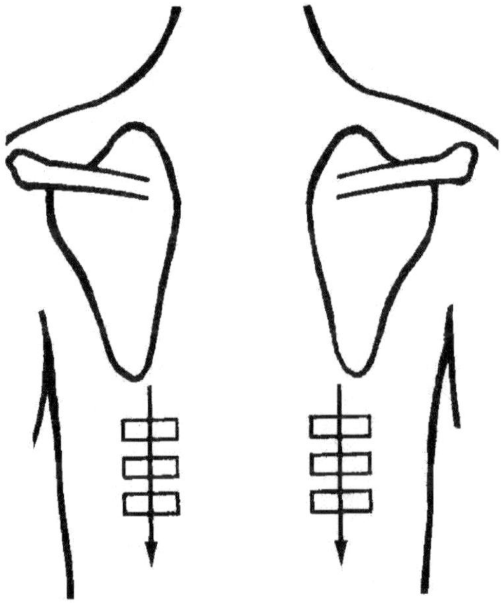

Figure 2-5. Diaphragm level.

2-7. PERCUSSION OF CHEST

To perform a percussion examination, strike the surface of the body. When this is done, various sounds can be heard. The sounds are different depending on the underlying structure of the body. There are two reasons to use percussion as an examination technique. First, percussion results in setting the chest wall and underlying tissues in motion. This produces sounds that can be heard. Second, percussion sounds can be divided into four recognizable notes. Train your ear to recognize the pitch and duration of these notes. The sound can indicate whether the underlying tissues are filled with air, filled with fluid, or solid. NOTE: Percussion will set tissues in motion only about five to seven centimeters into the chest, so the percussion examination technique is not a way to detect lesions that are very deep.

	Intensity	Pitch	Duration	Example Location
Flatness	soft	high	short	thigh
Dullness	medium	medium	medium	liver
Resonance	loud	low	long	normal lung
Tympany	loud	"musical timbre"		gastric air bubble or puffed out cheek

Table 2-1. Table of percussion notes.

a. **Procedure**. In order to perform the percussion examination technique, strike the stationary finger of one hand with a flexed finger of the other hand. The technique, described here, can be practiced on any surface. Here are the key points:

(1) Firmly rest the first joint of the middle finger of one hand on the patient's chest, but don't let the rest of the hand touch the chest (figure 2-5).

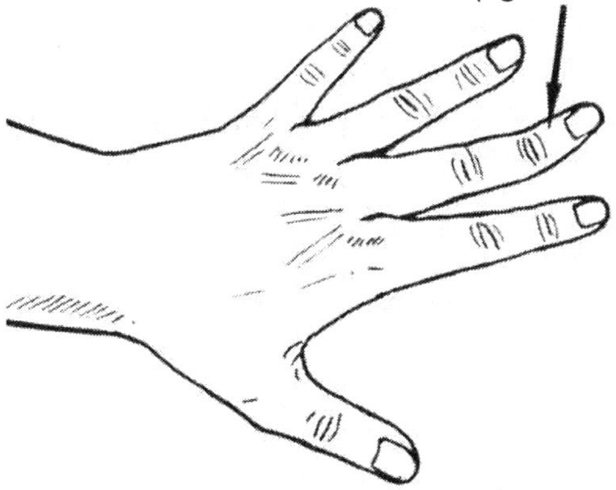

Figure 2-6. Hand and finger placement.

(2) Keep the fingers of the other hand flexed and the wrist loose (figure 2-7).

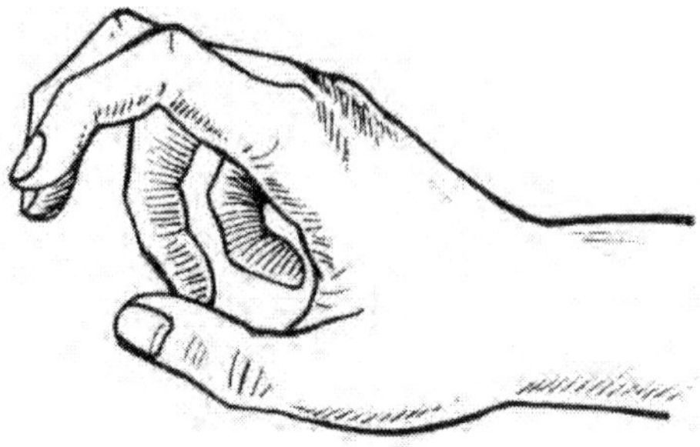

Figure 2-7. Hand position.

(3) With the tip of the middle finger of the flexed hand, strike the first joint of the middle finger of the hand that is on the patient's chest (figure 2-8). Have the motion come from the wrist.

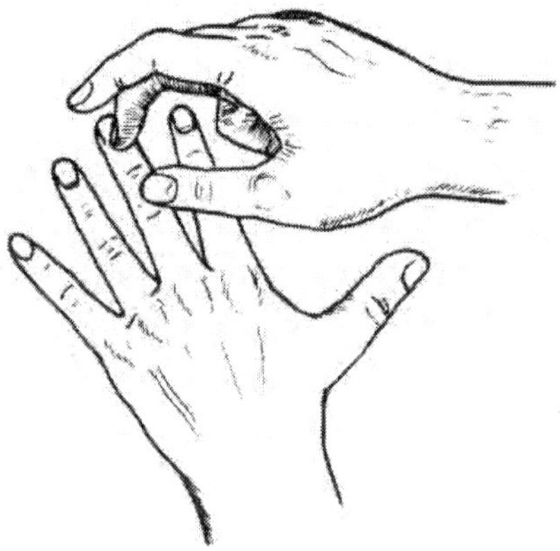

Figure 2-8. Striking position.

(4) Withdraw the striking finger immediately to avoid damping the vibration.

(5) Strike once or twice, then move your hands symmetrically to another part of the chest.

b. **Areas of Percussion**.

(1) Ideally, the patient should lie in the supine position (lying on the back, face upward) for percussion on the front of the chest. The patient should be sitting up for percussion on the back.

(2) If the patient is ill and unable to sit up, examine with the patient lying on the right or left side.

(3) Percuss the patient's anterior chest (figure 2-9). In a healthy patient, the entire upper chest is resonant except for the area of cardiac dullness. Percuss across the top of the body and work downward, symmetrically.

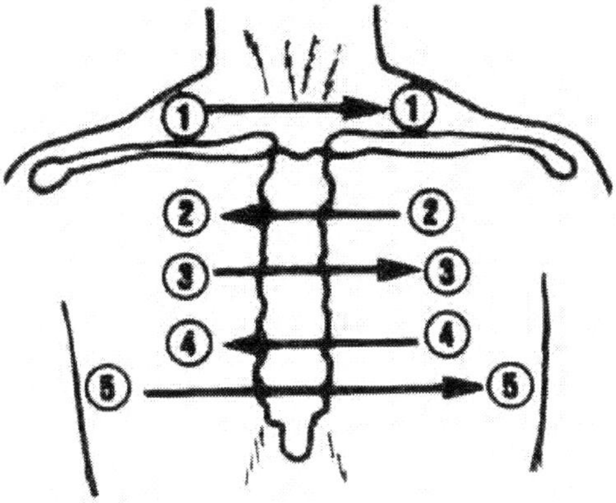

Figure 2-9. Anterior percussion.

(4) Percuss the patient's posterior chest, symmetrically down the chest wall making a side to side comparison (figure 2-10). Percussion over lung fields should reveal equal bilateral findings. Omit percussion over the shoulder blades.

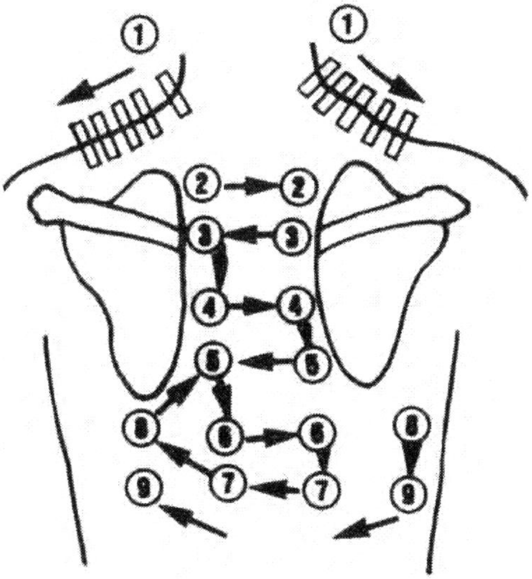

Figure 2-10. Posterior percussion.

(5) Measure the diaphragmatic excursion (movement of the diaphragm from a position of rest) by noting the difference between the levels of dullness when the person inhales fully and exhales fully. See figure 2-11. The difference is normally about 5 or 6 cm.

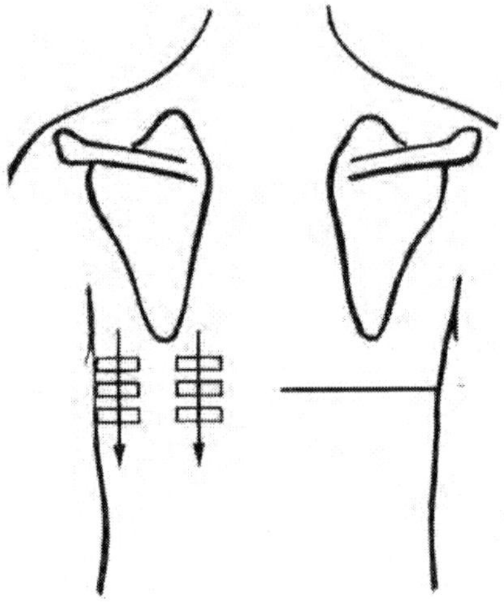

Figure 2-11. Diaphragmatic excursion.

2-8. AUSCULTATION OF CHEST

Auscultation (listening with a stethoscope) of the lungs is useful in estimating the airflow through the tracheobronchial tree, detecting an obstruction, and assessing the condition of the surrounding lungs and the pleural space.

a. Position the patient. Have the patient sitting or in a supine position. When the patient is lying down, examine his back by turning the patient from side to side.

b. Show the patient how you want him to breath through the mouth, deeper and more forcefully than usual.

c. Listen with the stethoscope.

(1) Start at the top of the back and work downward, comparing the right and the left sides.

(2) Then, start at the top of the chest and work downward, comparing symmetric points sequentially.

(a) Listen to one full breath in each location.

(b) Be alert for patient discomfort--light-headedness, faintness--that signals hyperventilation.

d. Auscultate normal breath sounds. Auscultate (examine by listening) normal breath sounds in accordance with table in 2-2.

NOTE: Two normal breath sounds can be auscultated as follows:

	Duration of inspiration and expiration	Pitch of expiration	Intensity of expiration	Sample location
vesicular breath sounds	inspiration greater than expiration	low	soft	most of lungs
bronchial or tubular breath sounds	expiration greater than inspiration	high	usually loud	over the trachea

Table 2-2. Auscultated normal breath sounds.

e. Auscultate vesicular breath sounds. These sounds are normally heard over the entire lung surface, except beneath the manubrium sterni and in the interscapular region. The sounds are long when the patient inhales and short when the patient exhales.

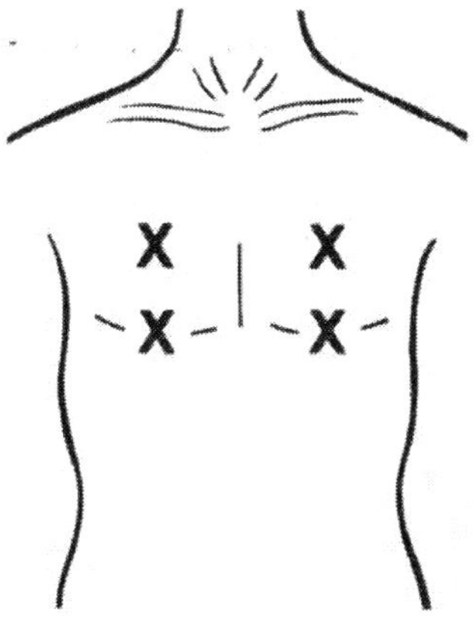

Figure 2-12. Auscultation over lung surfaces.

f. Auscultate bronchial (tubular) breath sounds. These sounds result from consolidation or compression of the pulmonary tissue that assists in the transmission of sound from the bronchial tree. Bronchial breath sounds do not occur in the normal lung except directly over the trachea. These sounds are short when the person breathes in and long when the person breathes out. The sounds are usually louder than vesicular breath sounds.

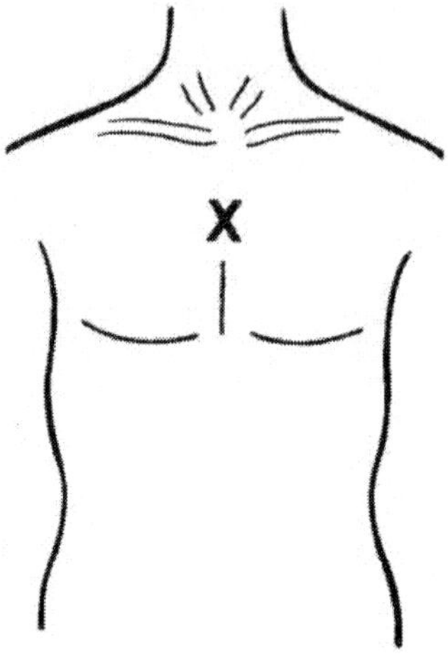

Figure 2-13. Auscultation over the trachea.

g. Check for abnormal sounds. Check for sounds in the lungs that are not modifications of breath or voice.

(1) Rhonchi. These are coarse, rattling sounds produced when the patient exhales. The sounds are usually very clear but might change with coughing. Low-pitched, these sounds occur when there is mucus in the bronchi.

(2) Rales (Crackles). Rales, also called crackles, are fine, rattling sounds. These are noncontinuous, high-pitched, fine crackles, like the sound of carbonated beverages. The sounds are usually heard when the patient breathes in and sometimes when the patient begins to exhale. These sounds are usually caused by the presence of fluid in the alveoli and the bronchioles. Sometimes the fluid is in these parts of the respiratory system, and sometimes the fluid is not there. This is the reason that sometimes the fine rattling can be heard, and sometimes it is not heard. Coughing usually makes the sounds louder.

(3) Wheezes. Wheezes are musical sounds like the high-pitched notes on a clarinet. Wheezes are produced by constricted or partially obstructed airways. The sounds can be heard when the patient breathes in.

(4) Pleural friction rub. These are scratchy sounds like crinkling Saran™ wrap. The sounds are produced by the movement of inflamed pleural surfaces rubbing together.

Continue with Exercises

EXERCISES, LESSON 2

INSTRUCTIONS. Answer these exercises by writing the answer in the space provided. After you have answered all the exercises, turn to "Solutions to Exercises" at the end of the lesson and check your answers.

1. The four techniques used in examining a patient are:

   a. ______________________________.

   b. ______________________________.

   c. ______________________________.

   d. ______________________________.

2. The patient's respiration rate should be _____to _____ breaths per minute.

3. List three things to observe when you are inspecting the patient.

   a. ______________________________.

   b. ______________________________.

   c. ______________________________.

4. When you are inspecting a patient, look at the skin and check for ___________

   and ___________________________.

5. During an inspection examination, observe the chest to see if it is shaped

   ________________________________.

6. List four uses of palpation of the chest.

   a. ______________________________________.

   b. ______________________________________.

   c. ______________________________________.

   d. ______________________________________.

7. During palpation, your fingers should not ____________________________.

8. When you are performing a palpation examination, it is normal to find that the

   __________________ side of the diaphragm is slightly higher than the

   ___________________________side.

9. List two reasons to perform chest percussion.

   a. ______________________________________.

   b. ______________________________________.

10. List two uses of examination of the chest by auscultation.

    a. ______________________________________.

    b. ______________________________________.

11. Coarse rattling sounds produced when the patient coughs are called

    ____.

12. Musical sounds like the high-pitched coughs are called ________________.

Check Your Answers on Next Page

SOLUTIONS TO EXERCISES, LESSON 2

1. Inspection.
   Palpation.
   Percussion.
   Auscultation. (para 2-4)

2. 12 to 20 (para 2-5b(1))

3. Respiration rate.
   Rhythm of breathing.
   Effort of breathing. (paras 2-5b(1)-(3))

4. Bruises and lacerations. (para 2-5c)

5. Symmetrically. (para 2-5d)

6. Identify areas of tenderness.
   Assess observed abnormalities.
   Further assess respiratory system.
   Elicit tactile fremitus. (paras 2-6a(1)-(4))

7. Move over the skin surface. (para 2-6b)

8. Right; left. (para 2-6f)

9. Set the chest wall and underlying tissues in motion to produce sounds that can be heard.

   These sounds can be used to help decide if the underlying tissues are filled with air, fluid, or a solid. (para 2-7)

10. You are correct if you listed any two of the following:

    Estimating airflow through the tracheobronchial tree.
    Detecting an obstruction.
    Assessing condition of the lungs and pleural space. (para 2-8)

11. Rhonchi. (para 2-8g(1))

12. Wheezes. (para 2-8g(3))

End of Lesson 2

LESSON ASSIGNMENT

LESSON 3 Infectious Respiratory Diseases.

LESSON ASSIGNMENT Paragraphs 3-1 through 3-15.

LESSON OBJECTIVES After completing this lesson, you should be able to:

3-1. Identify the characteristics, signs/symptoms, and treatment for these upper respiratory diseases: allergic rhinitis; paranasal sinusitis; common cold; acute pharyngitis; acute tonsillitis/strep throat.

3-2. Identify the characteristics, signs/symptoms, and treatment for these upper respiratory diseases with systemic effects: mononucleosis; influenza.

3-3. Identify the characteristics, signs/symptoms, and treatment for these types of pneumonia: staphylococcal pneumonia; mycoplasmal pneumonia; viral pneumonia; bronchial pneumonia.

SUGGESTION After completing the assignment, complete the exercises at the end of this lesson. These exercises will help you to achieve the lesson objectives.

LESSON 3

INFECTIOUS RESPIRATORY DISEASES

Section I. UPPER RESPIRATORY DISEASES

3-1. ALLERGIC RHINITIS.

a. **Definition/Characteristics**. Allergic rhinitis may be defined as the inflammation of nasal mucosa brought about by airborne pollens that react to release histamine. In other words, when some people breathe pollens that are in the air, the pollens cause histamine to be released. The excess of histamine in the body causes nasal mucosa to become inflamed. Causes of allergic rhinitis, more common during the warmest months of the year, include hay fever and allergic disorders which are common during seasons when the pollen count is high. Allergicrhinitis is also caused by house dust, occupational dust, molds, and animal danders (feathers, wool in blankets). Certain foods and drugs cause allergic rhinitis symptoms; sometimes bacteria causes this problem.

b. **Signs/Symptoms.**

(1) Nasal congestion.

(2) Profuse watery discharge.

(3) Itching of nose and conjunctiva.

(4) Sneezing.

c. **Treatment.** Treatment may include a combination of antihistamines, decongestants, or desensitization as well as management. Elimination of house dust, pollens, etc. may bring relief to the patient's symptoms.

(1) Antihistamines. For the majority of patients, antihistamines will not only control the symptoms of allergic rhinitis but also dry out the membranes. Caution: Antihistamines cause some persons to be sedated, depressed, sleepy, or uncoordinated. Watch for these reactions.

(2) Decongestants. Give decongestants if the patient suffers from nasal obstruction. Decongestants are effective for short-term but not long-term treatment.

(3) Desensitization. Several months before the season when the individual becomes acutely uncomfortable from pollen, give injections of pollen extracts that are specifically made for the individual. Continue giving the injections once a week during the peak of the pollen season.

3-2. PARANASAL SINUSITIS

a. **Definition/Characteristics.** Paranasal sinusitis is an infection of the mucous membranes that line the paranasal sinuses. Since the membrane that lines these sinuses is continuous with that of the of the nose and throat, paranasal sinusitis is a common complication of any upper respiratory infection. Causes of paranasal sinusitis include viruses, streptococci, and pneumococci.

b. **Signs/Symptoms.** Signs and symptoms of acute paranasal sinusitis are like those of acute rhinitis but are more severe. Included are headache, worse during the day; facial and tooth pain; tenderness over the sinuses; and fever and chills. There may be chronic recurrences of these signs and symptoms along with postnasal drip.

c. **Treatment.** The goals of treatment are to improve drainage and control infection. Vasoconstrictors such as steam inhalation and phenylephrine 0.25 percent spray used three times a day for a maximum of seven days may be used to open the nasal passages. In the case of acute paranasal sinusitis, antibiotics may be given. The drug of choice is penicillin G. If the patient is allergic to penicillin, erythromycin is an alternative drug. Patients suffering from chronic paranasal sinusitis may be given ampicillin or tetracycline.

d. **Complications.** Possible complications from paranasal sinusitis include osteomyelitis (inflammation of the bone marrow); meningitis (inflammation of the membranes covering the brain and spinal cord); and abscess.

3-3. COMMON COLD

a. **Definition/Characteristics.** The common cold is a contagious, viral infection of the upper respiratory tract. The cold is usually caused by a strain of rhinovirus. Over ninety distinct strains of rhinovirus are known to cause the common cold. Although not everyone is susceptible to infection from a cold virus, this respiratory infection occurs more often than all other diseases combined. Whether or not a person develops a cold after being exposed to a cold virus is determined to some extent by the person's general health. Fatigue, chilling of the body, wearing wet clothes and shoes, and the presence of irritating substances in the air make it more likely that the person will develop a cold.

b. **Signs/Symptoms.** These are signs and symptoms of the common cold:

(1) Malaise (general feeling of being unwell).

(2) Fever/chills.

(3) Headache.

(4) Nasal discomfort.

(5) Dry, sore throat.

(6) Cough (either productive or nonproductive).

(7) Mild leukocytosis (temporary increase in number of leukocytes in the blood).

c. **Treatment.** The patient should rest, drink fluids, take analgesics for pain, and use nasal decongestants for stuffiness in the nasal passages.

3-4. ACUTE PHARYNGITIS

a. **Definition/Characteristics.** Acute pharyngitis is an inflammation of the pharynx. This disease, inflammation of the mucosa of the pharynx, usually occurs as part of an upper respiratory tract disorder. The nose, sinuses, larynx, and trachea may also be affected. The most common causes are bacterial or viral infection. Very rarely, acute pharyngitis is caused by inhalation of irritant gases or ingestion of irritant liquids. Sometimes, acute pharyngitis is one symptom of a specific disease such as measles, chickenpox, scarlet fever, or whooping cough.

b. **Signs/Symptoms.** Common signs and symptoms are listed below. A complication may be a secondary infection.

(1) Dry and sore throat.

(2) Fever.

(3) Malaise.

(4) Strep infection may be present with white pus pocket formation.

(5) Cough.

c. **Treatment.** Rest, light diet, analgesics for pain, and nonirritating gargles (saline) should relieve the symptoms. Give antibiotics for initial or complicating bacterial infection.

3-5. ACUTE TONSILLITIS/STREP THROAT

a. **Definition/Characteristics.**

(1) Tonsillitis. Tonsillitis is a painful disease caused by bacteria or viruses that infect one or both of the palatine tonsils. People between the ages of ten and forty have the majority of tonsillitis attacks.

(2) Strep throat. Strep throat is an infectious disease that affects the membranes of the throat and tonsils. This disease is also called septic sore throat, acute streptococcal pharyngitis, and acute streptococcal tonsillitis. The disease is caused by group A beta-hemolytic streptococci bacteria. It spreads from person to person through droplets of moisture sprayed from the nose and mouth. Some people only carry the bacteria. These carriers exhibit no symptoms themselves but spread the disease.

b. **Signs/Symptoms.**

(1) Sore throat.

(2) Strong breath odor.

(3) Pain in swallowing.

(4) Fever/chills.

(5) Posterior cervical lymphadenopathy (disease of the lymph nodes).

(6) Headache.

(7) Malaise.

(8) Red or swollen tonsils or pharynx (with or without fluid, cells, or cellular debris from blood vessels (exudates)).

(9) Increased white blood cells with bacterial pharyngitis.

(10) With bacterial pharyngitis (strep throat), the throat culture is positive.

c. **Complications.** Chronic tonsillitis, acute otitis media (accumulation of fluid in the middle ear), and acute sinusitis are complications which may occur as a result of tonsillitis or strep throat.

d. **Treatment.** Treatment includes rest, fluids, light diet, saline (salt water) gargles, and analgesics for pain. If indicated, prescribe antibiotics as follows:

(1) Penicillin VK 250 mg, 1 tablet by mouth 6 times a day for 10 days.

(2) An alternate drug is erythromycin in the dosage of 250 mg. Take 1 tablet by mouth 6 times a day for 10 days.

(3) If the patient has difficulty swallowing, give benzathine penicillin G (bicillin), 1.2 million units intramuscularly.

Section II. UPPER RESPIRATORY DISEASES WITH SYSTEMIC EFFECTS

3-6. MONONUCLEOSIS

a. **Definition/Characteristics.** Characterized by the presence of more than the normal number of mononuclear leukocytes in the blood, mononucleosis gets its name from these mononuclear (single nucleus) cells. Although this disease occurs mostly in young adults, children and older people do sometimes contract mononucleosis. One of the herpes viruses, the Epstein-Barr virus, is the cause, and direct contact between people--kissing, for example--can spread the disease. A simple blood test can determine whether a person has mononucleosis. Some sheep's blood is mixed with a sample of clear liquid of the patient's blood. If the patient has mononucleosis, the sheep's blood cells will stick to one another.

b. **Signs/Symptoms.** The following signs and symptoms may be present:

(1) Fever.

(2) Malaise.

(3) Sore throat.

(4) Hepatic (liver) dysfunction.

(5) Lymphadenopathy (may cause lymph node enlargement).

(6) Hepatosplenomelegaly (enlargement of the liver and spleen).

(7) Abnormal lymphocytes.

(8) Marked asthenia (weakness).

c. **Treatment.** There is no specific treatment for mononucleosis. Generally, rest and nourishment are prescribed. Specific symptoms are treated; for example, saline gargles for sore throat and analgesics for pain. Secondary infections are treated with appropriate antibiotics. Strenuous activities should be avoided.

d. **Precautions.** The symptoms of hepatitis and respiratory occlusion are treated. If the spleen ruptures, emergency removal of the spleen may be necessary.

3-7. INFLUENZA

a. **Definition/Characteristics.** Influenza is a highly contagious disease caused by a virus. The disease spreads by an infected person exhaling the virus, which is then breathed in by an uninfected person. Once inhaled, the virus comes in contact with cells of the upper air passages, and new influenza viruses are released in the body. These viruses infect other cells along the respiratory tract sometimes spreading deep within the lungs and to other parts of the body. The formerly healthy person exhales viruses that may be carried away by the air to be inhaled by someone else. Several different strains of virus including A, B, C, and swine viruses infect people. When the body produces substances called antibodies, people develop immunity or resistance to influenza. The antibodies attach themselves to influenza viruses and prevent the viruses from infecting cells. It is possible for the virus to change its chemical composition so that the antibodies no longer work. Then, the cells of the body must form new antibodies.

b. **Signs/Symptoms.** The onset of signs and symptoms is usually sudden and can include the following:

(1) Slight fever lasting 1 to 7 days (usually 3 to 5 days).

(2) Cough which is nonproductive and dry, occurring in spasms.

(3) Headache.

(4) Nasal stuffiness and discharge.

(5) Mildly infected throat.

(6) Chills.

(7) Myalgia (pain in muscles).

(8) Occasional nausea, diarrhea.

c. **Complications.** These complications can occur:

(1) Necrosis of the respiratory epithelium (tissue death of linings in the respiratory system) which makes a secondary bacterial infection possible.

(2) The most common complication is pneumococcal pneumonia.

(3) The most serious complication is a staphylococcal infection.

d. **Diagnosis.** Isolation of the virus from throat washing or sputum allows a diagnosis of influenza.

e. **Treatment.** Bed rest is of great importance in order to prevent complications. Analgesics can be taken for muscle pain and headache. The patient should drink plenty of fluids. Antibiotics may be given for secondary bacterial infections.

f. **Prevention.** Flu vaccine is available for vaccination of the general population.

Section III. LOWER RESPIRATORY DISEASES

3-8. ACUTE BRONCHITIS

a. **Definition/Characteristics.** Acute bronchitis is inflammation of the bronchial mucous membrane of the bronchial tree. Infection, dust, chemical agents, and/or allergies can cause bronchitis. When the bronchi are infected, the mucous membranes (linings) of the bronchi secrete mucus and pus cells (white blood cells that can attack infectious agents). The large outpouring of mucus partially obstructs the airways. Additionally, the irritated membranes may swell, further obstructing the airways.

b. **Signs/Symptoms.**

(1) Chilliness.

(2) Malaise.

(3) Soreness and constriction behind the sternum-worse when patient coughs.

(4) Slight fever.

(5) Cough, at first dry and painful; later, green or yellowish sputum with pus cells.

c. **Treatment.** Treatment should include bed rest and increased fluid intake. Medication to reduce the fever and pain can be taken. Antibiotics can be used, if indicated. Steam inhalation can open air passages.

3-9. PLEURITIS

a. **Definition/Characteristics.** Pleuritis is an inflammation of the pleural lining, a lining that covers the lungs and the chest cavity. The two surfaces of this lining are moist and allow the lungs to move smoothly over the chest wall when a person breathes. The surfaces of the lining become dry and rough and rub together when the pleura lining is inflamed. This condition, called pleurisy or pleuritis, is very painful and becomes more painful when the person breathes deeply or coughs. Most cases of pleuritis occur as complications of some other respiratory condition such as pneumonia, tuberculosis, or another infectious disease. The underlying disease must be treated in order to cure the pleuritis.

b. **Signs/Symptoms.** Pleuritis signs and symptoms include the following:

(1) Pain--varies from vague discomfort to sharp severe stabbing in the chest. The pain becomes worse when the person coughs or breathes deeply.

(2) Respirations--short, shallow, and rapid.

(3) Motion--limited on the affected side.

(4) Breath--diminished sound.

(5) Fever.

(6) Chills.

(7) Friction rub--usually heard only after 24 to 48 hours.

c. **Treatment.** The patient should rest in bed, use heat on the area that is painful, and take analgesics for fever and mild pain.

3-10. PNEUMONIA

a. **Characteristics/Definition.** Pneumonia is an acute infection of the alveoli spaces of the lungs. Causes of pneumonia include injury to the respiratory mucosa with pneumonia as a secondary infection, influenza, common colds, and bronchitis. There are three types of pneumonia: bacterial; mycoplasmal (bacteria having no cell wall and bounded by a triple-layered membrane); viral. Bacterial pneumonia is further subdivided into these types: pneumococcal; staphylococcal; klebsiella (Friedlander's bacillus); streptococcal; and influenza bacillus.

b. **Pneumococcal Pneumonia.** Sixty to eighty percent of bacterial pneumonia cases are pneumococcal pneumonia. This type of pneumonia, an inflammation of the lung tissue, is probably caused by a lowering of a person's natural resistance to infection. These conditions can lower a person's resistance to this type of pneumonia:

viral respiratory diseases; malnutrition; exposure to cold; noxious gases; and alcoholic intoxication.

(1) Signs/Symptoms.

(a) Mild nasopharyngitis (inflammation of the nasopharynx)-- several days before onset of the disease.

(b) Sudden onset of illness.

(c) Vomiting.

(d) Severe chest pain--in 70 percent of the cases.

(e) Productive cough--rusty sputum.

(f) Fever (103 - 106°F)/chills.

(g) Often acutely ill.

(h) Dyspnea (labored breathing) and cyanosis. Cyanosis in light-skinned individuals gives a bluish cast to skin, lips, and nail beds. In dark-skinned individuals or blacks, the discoloration is grey or grayish. The cause is not enough oxygen in the blood.

(i) Decreased movement on one side of the chest.

(j) Severe, shaking chill.

(k) Signs of consolidation (inflammatory solidification of the lung); dull to percussion; bronchial breath sounds; fine rales.

(l) Gram-positive diplococci (bacterium which has not separated but occurs in pairs as a result of disease).

(m) Blood culture positive.

(n) Chest x-ray--originally may show vague haziness but later shows shadows in area of lung involvement.

(2) Course. Fever and symptoms subside dramatically within 72 hours after the start of the antibiotics in over fifty percent of the patients. When the patient begins to get better, the fine rales and tubular breathing become coarse, sticky rales. If the patient experiences pseudocrisis (the fever subsides, but the other symptoms continue), watch for shock.

(3) Treatment.

(a) The drug of choice is penicillin given by intramuscular injection. The dosage ranges from 600,000 units of procaine penicillin every 12 hours if the illness is moderate to 1 million units of aqueous penicillin G given every 4 hours in an intravenous infusion for a patient seriously ill. Continue penicillin treatment 72 hours after the patient's temperature has returned to normal. If the patient is allergic to penicillin, administer tetracycline or erythromycin.

(b) The patient should have bed rest, oxygen, fluids, and electrolytes. In two to three weeks, the patient should have a follow-up chest x-ray.

(4) Prognosis. In treated groups, there is 95 percent recovery. In groups of people who are untreated, 20 to 40 percent do not survive (usually in the under 2 and over 45 age groups).

Section IV. OTHER CAUSES OF PNEUMONIA

3-11. INTRODUCTION

Other causes of pneumonia include other bacteria, viruses, mycoplasmas, pulmonary embolus, and atelectasis. The physical findings and x-ray evidence may be similar. In order to treat a pneumonia case properly, it is important to determine the cause by blood culture and sputum examination. Occasionally, other methods may be necessary to determine the cause.

3-12. STAPHYLOCOCCAL PNEUMONIA

a. **Predisposing Factors.** A person with a respiratory tract viral infection can contract this type of pneumonia. A debilitated patient such as a postsurgical patient also may contract staphylococcal pneumonia.

b. **Signs/Symptoms.** Signs of consolidation (dullness and tubular breathing) are infrequent, but pleural effusion (liquid in the pleural space) is common. Gram-positive cocci (bacterial cells) help confirm that the patient has staphylococcal pneumonia.

c. **Treatment.** Initial treatment consists of a vigorous antibiotic which should be a penicillin derivative other than penicillin G or ampicillin. If the patient is sensitive to penicillin, the next drug of choice would be cephalothin given for 8 to 14 days and administered intravenously or vancomycin twice a day administered intravenously.

d. **Prognosis.** There is a 15 to 20 percent mortality. Whether or not the patient recovers depends on his underlying general health and the effect of the drug administered on the virus.

3-13. MYCOPLASMAL PNEUMONIA

Mycoplasmas can be defined as bacteria that do not have a cell wall. Mycoplasma pneumonia is a respiratory, disease-producing microorganism that occurs from time to time and spreads in groups of people--the family, school populations, the military.

a. **Signs/Symptoms.**

(1) Slow onset of headache and malaise.

(2) Cough, nonproductive or a small amount.

(3) Not acutely ill.

(4) No cyanosis or dyspnea.

(5) Only mild signs of consolidation.

(6) Shadows on the chest x-ray.

(7) White blood count is normal.

(8) Gram stain shows normal flora (flora-normal bacteria in intestine).

(9) Frequently affects families.

(10) Generally, limits itself.

(11) Cold agglutinins positive (50 percent or more).

b. **Treatment.** Follow the same general measures as for pneumococcal pneumonia. Antimicrobial drugs are not necessary in mild or moderate cases of this disease. In severe cases, tetracycline or erythromycin may be given for two or three weeks.

3-14. VIRAL PNEUMONIA

Viral pneumonia may be caused by the adenoviruses (a group of DNA viruses, some of which can cause respiratory tract infections), respiratory viruses, the parainfluenza viruses, and probably other viruses not yet identified with viral pneumonia. It is difficult to distinguish viral pneumonia from primary atypical pneumonia on the basis of physical and x-ray findings. It is necessary to examine sputum by Gram's stain and culture to diagnose viral pneumonia.

a. **Signs/Symptoms.** The onset of viral pneumonia is usually slow and occurs after an upper respiratory infection. The disease is similar to mycoplasmal pneumonia except that the illness is shorter and cold agglutinins and lymphocytosis are negative. The disease, however, is dangerous to two groups of people: debilitated persons with chronic pulmonary or cardiac disease and infants under six months. For these patients, the disease is rapid and often fatal. The signs of the disease are much like those for pneumococcal pneumonia. Other signs and symptoms for persons not in these two high risk groups include:

(1) Mild rales.

(2) Nonproductive cough.

(3) Mild illness.

(4) Abnormal chest x-ray, rarely.

b. **Treatment.** Treatment is supportive in that the symptoms should be treated. No antibiotics are given.

3-15. BRONCHIAL PNEUMONIA

Bronchial pneumonia is an infection of the alveolar spaces of the respiratory bronchiole.

a. **Signs/Symptoms.** Bronchial pneumonia begins slowly, often after a person has had an upper respiratory infection. The patient may cough and spit out a greenish, yellowish sputum. The patient's chest may be congested and feel tight, yet a percussion examination will be normal. Auscultation indicates the patient has scattered rhonchi, usually on both sides of the chest. His respiration, pulse, and temperature will be above normal.

b. **Treatment.** Treat the symptoms of the disease. Specific problems can be treated with drugs. A patient with mycoplasmal pneumonia can be given tetracycline. Administer penicillin to patients with either pneumococcal or streptoccal pneumonia. If the patient has gram-negative rods, administer streptomycin.

Continue with Exercises

EXERCISES, LESSON 3

INSTRUCTIONS. Answer these exercises by writing the answer in the space provided. After you have answered all the exercises, turn to "Solutions to Exercises" at the end of the lesson and check your answers.

1. Fever and chills, facial and tooth pain, and a headache which is worse during the day are symptoms of ______________________________.

2. Acute pharyngitis is sometimes a symptom of a specific disease such as measles, ________________________, whooping cough, or chickenpox.

3. Abnormal lymphocytes, lymph node disease, and hepatic dysfunction are symptoms of ______________________________.

4. ___________________________, an inflammation of the lining which covers the lungs and chest cavity, is usually a complication of some other respiratory condition such as pneumonia or tuberculosis.

5. Acute bronchitis can be caused by dust, chemical agents and/or ____________ to pollens.

6. Three types of pneumonia are bacterial pneumonia,__________________ pneumonia, and viral pneumonia.

7. When the patient breathes in airborne pollen, his nasal passages become inflamed. He is suffering from __________________________________.

8. A patient with an increased white blood cell count, pain on swallowing, and strong breath odor could have strep throat or ________________________.

9. A highly contagious disease caused by a virus whose strains include A, B, and C is ______________________________________.

10. Nasal congestion, profuse watery discharge, itching of nose and conjunctiva, and sneezing are all signs and symptoms of ______________________________.

11. Paranasal sinusitis is ____

____

12. There are over ninety distinct strains of __________________________ that can cause the common cold.

13. The most common causes of acute pharyngitis are bacterial infection or ______________________________________.

14. Septic sore throat and acute streptococcal pharyngitis are other names for the respiratory infection commonly called _____________________________.

15. The respiratory disease which gets its name from the abnormal increase in single nucleus cells in the body is _________________________.

16. Influenza is a highly contagious disease which is caused by _______________.

17. A person with pleuritis most likely has some other respiratory condition such as _____________________, ________________, or another infectious disease.

18. Mild rales, nonproductive cough, and ________________ are signs and symptoms of viral pneumonia.

Check Your Answers on Next Page

SOLUTIONS TO EXERCISES, LESSON 3

1. Paranasal sinusitis. (para 3-2b(1)(a)-(d))

2. Scarlet fever. (para 3-4a)

3. Mononucleosis. (para 3-6b)

4. Pleuritis. (para 3-9)

5. Allergies. (para 3-8a)

6. Mycoplasmal. (para 3-10a)

7. Allergic rhinitis. (para 3-1a)

8. Tonsillitis. (para 3-5b)

9. Influenza. (para 3-7a)

10. Allergic rhinitis. (para 3-1b)

11. Paranasal sinusitis is <u>an</u> infection of the mucous membranes which line the paranasal sinuses or the bony framework of the sinuses. (para 3-2a)

12. Rhinovirus. (para 3-3a)

13. Viral infection. (para 3-4a)

14. Strep throat. (para 3-5a(2))

15. Mononucleosis. (para 3-6a)

16. A virus. (para 3-7a)

17. Pneumonia, tuberculosis. (para 3-9a)

18. Mild illness. (para 3-14a)

End of Lesson 3

LESSON ASSIGNMENT

LESSON 4 Chronic Obstructive Pulmonary Diseases.

TEXT ASSIGNMENT Paragraphs 4-1 through 4-10.

LESSON OBJECTIVES After completing this lesson, you should be able to:

4-1. Identify the characteristics, signs/symptoms, and treatment for asthma.

4-2. Identify the characteristics, signs/symptoms, and treatment for chronic bronchitis.

4-3. Identify the characteristics, signs/symptoms, and treatment for emphysema.

SUGGESTION After completing the assignment, complete the exercises at the end of this lesson. These exercises will help you to achieve the lesson objectives.

CHRONIC OBSTRUCTIVE PULMONARY DISEASES

Section I. ASTHMA

4-1. DEFINITION/CHARACTERISTICS

a. Chronic obstructive pulmonary diseases (COPD) affect one out of five Americans. Asthma and bronchitis are common forms of COPD and are found more often in men than in women. The incidence of these diseases is more common among cigarette smokers than people who do not smoke. Asthma is a disease characterized by attacks of wheezing and difficult breathing. Spasms of the smooth muscles that lie in the walls of the smaller bronchi and bronchioles bring on the attacks and cause these passageways to close partially. Asthma can be caused by environmental factors such as dust or cold air. Asthma can also be caused by an infection, exercise, or emotional upset.

b. In an asthma attack, several bodily changes make it difficult for air to go through bronchi passageways. These changes include bronchoconstriction (bronchial muscles constricting), mucus secretion in the bronchi, and edema (fluid retention) in the bronchial wall. The difficulty in bringing air through those passages accounts for a sign almost always associated with asthma--wheezing.

c. There are five types of asthma. They are:

(1) Extrinsic (allergic) asthma.

(2) Intrinsic asthma.

(3) Triad asthma.

(4) Nasal polyp asthma.

(5) Bronchospasm.

4-2. SIGNS/SYMPTOMS

a. **Extrinsic (allergic) Asthma.** This type of asthma usually affects children and young adults who have a personal or family history of being hypersensitive to substances in the environment, foods, or air substances that are inhaled. An individual can inherit an allergy to drugs, vaccines, and anesthetic agents also.

(1) Inhalant allergens include:

(a) Pollens.

(b) Dusts.

(c) Animal danders/hairs.

(d) Feathers.

(e) Molds.

(2) Food allergens include:

(a) Milk.

(b) Eggs.

(c) Nuts.

(d) Chocolate.

(e) Fish.

(f) Shellfish

(g) Strawberries.

(3) Irritant inhalants include:

(a) Fumes.

(b) Cold air.

(c) Air pollutants.

b. **Intrinsic Asthma.** This type of asthma is more common among adults over 35, especially women. Upper and lower respiratory tract infections may cause intrinsic asthma even though there has been no family or childhood history of the disease.

c. **Triad Asthma.** As the name implies, triad asthma includes three elements at the same time: aspirin (ASA), indomethacin (Indocin), and yellow food dye.

(1) Signs/symptoms of triad asthma include:

(a) Respiratory distress.

(b) Cough.

(c) Flushing--redness of skin.

(d) Cyanosis--blueness or grayishness of skin from oxygen poor blood.

(e) Apprehension.

(f) Tachycardia (rapid pulse).

(g) Perspiration.

(h) Flaring of nasal alae (outer side of each nostril).

(i) Dyspnea--labored or difficult breathing.

(j) Wheezing--quite audible or absent.

(2) The patient may have difficulty breathing and exhibiting these signs of respiratory distress:

(a) Dyspnea.

(b) Wheezing.

(c) Hyperresonance--very loud body sounds.

(d) Rhonchi.

(e) Wheezing in a particular part of the body indicating an obstruction by a foreign body or a tumor in the area. If a patient is wheezing, it is not safe to say that the patient has asthma. <u>Not every person who wheezes has asthma</u>. Wheezing may also be caused by:

<u>1</u> Acute left heart failure (cardiac asthma).

<u>2</u> Smoke inhalation.

3 Chronic bronchitis.

4 Acute pulmonary embolism.

4-3. LABORATORY FINDINGS

a. Chest x-rays usually show nothing abnormal.

b. If the patient shows signs of wheezing and dyspnea, chest x-rays and other laboratory tests are used to rule out the following:

(1) Pneumothorax - an accumulation of air or gas in the pleural space.

(2) Mucus plugging - a glob of mucus obstructing passageways.

(3) Pneumonia.

(4) Foreign body - obstructing passageways.

(5) Cancer.

4-4. TREATMENT

a. **Purpose.** The purpose of treatment in an asthma attack is twofold. First, it is necessary to treat the symptoms of the attack. Then, causes of the attack should be diagnosed and treatment begun to prevent further attacks.

b. **Hospitalization**. Consider hospitalization when the patient has had one or more of the following situations:

(1) Seventy-two hours of unremitting asthma.

(2) One hour of adequate acute therapy without improvement.

(3) Three trips to the emergency room in three days.

(4) Quiet chest.

(5) Pulsus paradox--an abnormal decrease in systolic pressure during inspiration, the decrease being greater than 10 mm of mercury (Hg).

(6) Sternocleidomastoid muscle and intercostal muscle withdrawing.

(7) Low carbon dioxide pressure (PCO_2).

c. **Monitoring**. During treatment for an acute asthma attack, monitor arterial blood gases every 30 to 60 minutes.

d. **Long-Term Therapy.** Long-term therapy is an attempt to identify the cause of asthma attacks and prevent those causes. Long-term therapy includes:

(1) Discovering and avoiding, if possible, whatever causes the asthma attack.

(2) Being desensitized against whatever is causing the asthma; for example, desensitization against ragweed, other pollens, etc.

(3) Taking appropriate medication. Tedral, Quibron, aminophylline, and steroids are drugs that can be used to treat asthma.

e. **Asthma in Children.** The treatment for asthma in children requires providing a pleasant and understanding home environment. Over-protection or parental resentment must be avoided.

f. **Acute Asthma Attack.** An acute attack of asthma is treated as a respiratory emergency. First, determine what medications the patient has taken within the last 12 hours.

(1) Procedure for an adult patient is:

(a) Open the airway if it is not open.

(b) Give humidified oxygen or a nebulizer (a device for throwing a spray). Use an intermittent positive pressure breathing (PPB) device if one is available. Do not use the unmodified demand valve on the PPB device because the dry gases it will send to the airway makes the mucus secretions worse.

(c) Establish an IV with a solution of five percent water with dextrose (D5W) or D5/normal saline.

(d) Administer epinephrine 1:1000, 0.3 to 0.5 ml subcutaneously (adult dose)if the patient has not taken large doses of inhalant bronchodilators. Repeat the dose in thirty minutes, if necessary.

(e) Aminophylline may be given by adding 250 mg of the drug to a 250 ml bag of D5/W. This infusion can be attached to the IV in piggyback fashion.

(f) Bronchodilators such as epinephrine (Isoproterenol, Isuprel) or Isoetharine (Bronkosol)may be administered by aerosol.

WARNING

DO NOT give sedatives that may depress respiration or antihistamines that dry secretions.

DO NOT give aspirin. Many asthmatics are allergic to aspirin.

(2) Procedure for a child is:

(a) Give oxygen.

(b) The drug of choice is epinephrine, 1:1000 0.01 ml/kg to 0.3 ml is the maximum dosage. The dosage may be repeated once or twice every 20 minutes. Alternative drugs that may be used include the following:

1 Sus-Phrine (1:200 aqueous suspension of epinephrine).

2 Theophylline preparation administered in a 4 mg/kg of body weight IV in 25 cc D5W over 5-15 minutes not exceeding 25 mg per minute. IV hydration is important (D5W or D5-saline wide open).

(c) Avoid using sedatives and oral preparations when treating asthma in an emergency situation.

(d) Aminophylline suppositories are a possible treatment.

CAUTION: Administering epinephrine after the use of over the counter (OTC) bronchodilators can cause severe circulatory disease or cardiac arrhythmias.

(3) In the case of a prolonged asthma attack, consider that the cause might be an infection or an allergen.

(4) Status asthmaticus. This condition is considered a medical emergency. Status asthmaticus is a severe prolonged asthmatic attack that can't be broken with epinephrine.

(a) Signs/symptoms include the following:

1 Chest that is severely distended.

2 Severe dyspnea (difficult or labored breathing).

3 Prominent use of accessory muscles.

4 Breath sounds (wheezes may be entirely inaudible).

5 Exhaustion.

6 Severe acidosis (accumulation of acid or depletion of the alkaline reserve in the blood and body tissues).

7 Dehydration.

(b) Other signs/symptoms may be:

1 Hypoxia (lack of oxygen reaching body tissues) contributing to encephalopathy (disease of the brain or spinal cord).

2 Respiratory acidosis.

3 Pneumomediastinum (presence of air or gas in the mediastinum which may interfere with respiration and circulation).

4 Possible progressive respiratory tract impairment.

(c) Treatment. Treatment is similar to that for acute asthma and includes the following:

1 Give oxygen by intermittent positive pressure breathing (IPPB). A machine delivering IPPB forces oxygen into the patient as the patient starts to take a breath. The machine automatically forces enough oxygen into the patient's lungs to open the alveoli.

2 Administer sodium bicarbonate intravenously to counteract acidosis. If you must add the medication to the primary intravenous bottle, use strict aseptic technique and follow this basic procedure:

a Wash your hands.

b Check the medication order.

c Prepare the medication and draw it up in a syringe.

d Remove the metal protector and rubber diaphragm from the bottle.

e Insert the needle into the injection site.

f Mix the solution and medication.

g Label the bottle.

h Discard the used needle and syringe.

i Record the medication.

3 Reassure the patient.

4 Transport the patient to a hospital immediately.

5 Begin an IV lifeline of dextrose in water solution (D5W).

Section II. CHRONIC BRONCHITIS

4-5. DEFINITION/CHARACTERISTICS

Chronic bronchitis is an inflammation of the bronchi of long duration. There is a productive cough associated with recurring infections of the lower respiratory tract. The result is a reduced ability to ventilate (breathe in and out) the lungs. A characteristic is an excessive, recurrent, mucus-producing cough. The patient is usually a heavy cigarette smoker who is obese. The soft tissues around the patient's fingers and toes may have undergone changes, but not the bone structure.

4-6. SIGNS/SYMPTOMS

As the disease becomes more severe, these signs/symptoms may be noticed in the patient:

a. Rales--a dry or moist sound according to the absence or presence of fluids in the air passages.

b. Rhonchi--a dry, coarse sound in the bronchial tubes due to a partial obstruction.

c. Wheeze--a whistling sound made in breathing.

d. Light fever--101 to 102 degrees Fahrenheit.

e. Back and muscle pain.

f. Cyanosis (blue bloater)--bluish discoloration of the skin and/or membranes. In blacks and dark-skinned individuals, the skin discolors to gray or a grayish tone.

g. More purulent (containing pus) and increase in volume of mucus produced with a cough.

h. Patient weakened by hypoxia (lack of adequate oxygen).

i. Confusion due to hypoxia.

j. Muscle twitching.

k. Edema (abnormal accumulation of fluid in body tissues).

l. Jugular vein distention.

m. Barrel chest, perhaps.

n. Productive cough with sputum color changes.

4-7. TREATMENT

Keep in mind that the patient may be suffering from another disease, and bronchitis is a secondary problem. Then remember the following:

a. The patient should avoid possible irritants such as smoking, allergenic agents, fumes and/or other irritants.

b. Codeine phosphate or a comparable antitussive agent can be used to suppress a nonproductive cough.

c. Mist inhalations (cool or warmed) and adequate fluid intake can be used to cope with thick sputum.

d. A drug such as terbutaline can be used to relieve bronchial spasm (violent cough).

e. Antihistamine drugs may reduce bronchial inflammation due to allergy.

f. Other measures may be taken depending on the cause of the bronchitis.

Section III. EMPHYSEMA

4-8. DEFINITION/CHARACTERISTICS

The word emphysema means "blown up" or "full of air." In emphysema, the alveolar walls of the lungs have lost their elasticity causing air to remain trapped in the lungs when the person breathes out. A first symptom is that the person exhales less than his usual amount of air. Alveoli in other areas of the lungs become damaged later, and many alveoli may unite, thus further reducing the overall volume of air the person is able to inhale.

a. Eventually, the lungs become permanently inflated because they have lost their elasticity. The size of a person's chest increases to adjust to the new larger size of the permanently inflated lungs. At this point, the person has to work voluntarily to exhale. The oxygen in the blood is a little lowered, and the person becomes breathless from any mild exercise in which the blood cells need more oxygen. As the disease progresses, unusually high amounts of carbon dioxide dissolve in the plasma producing acid conditions that are toxic to brain cells. This causes the body's inspiration area to become less active which causes the respiration rate to slow down.

b. A number of factors can cause emphysema.

(1) A tendency in some families for chronic obstructive pulmonary diseases such as silicosis (a disease caused by inhaling stone, sand, or flint dust into the lungs)or fibrosis (formation of fibers in the lungs).

(2) A history of chronic bronchial obstruction such as bronchitis or asthma.

(3) Cigarette smoking is thought to be a major cause.

(4) The result of a penetrating wound of the chest wall.

4-9. SIGNS/SYMPTOMS

a. The signs and symptoms of emphysema are listed as follows:

(1) Shortness of breath.

(2) Pursed lip breathing (pink puffers).

(3) Barrel chest appearance.

(4) Wheezing.

(5) Chronic cough.

(6) Expectoration with small quantities of mucus.

(7) Dyspnea (difficult or labored breathing) on exertion.

(8) Hyperresonant to percussion.

(9) Appears thin and wasted (weight loss).

(10) Difficult to hear sounds in body by listening to lungs with stethoscope.

b. In all cases of chronic cough, asthma, or any disease that produces pulmonary fibrosis, a diagnosis of emphysema should be considered. Early diagnosis is difficult, but advanced cases of emphysema are evident by the following symptoms:

(1) Severe dyspnea (difficult or labored breathing).

(2) Distended chest.

(3) Depressed diaphragm.

(4) Abnormal blood gases.

4-10. TREATMENT

Treatment for emphysema is designed to correct or diminish the causes. For example, if air pollution, occupational exposure to industrial dust, or cigarette smoke is causing the problem, the patient must remove himself from these air pollutants as much as possible. Mist inhalations and supplemental fluids can be used to thin secretions that are thick. Other treatments designed to combat the cause of the condition can be used. Bed rest is not the main treatment but can be given when necessary.

Continue with Exercises

EXERCISES, LESSON 4

INSTRUCTIONS. Answer these exercises by writing the answer in the space provided or choosing the statement that best answers the question. After you have answered all the exercises, turn to "Solutions to Exercises" at the end of the lesson and check your answers.

1. Asthma and bronchitis are common forms of ______________________________

   ____

2. Asthma is a disease in which muscle spasms in the walls of the small bronchi and bronchioles bring on the attack and cause ______________________________

   ____.

3. List the five types of asthma.

   a. ______________________________.

   b. ______________________________.

   c. ______________________________.

   d. ______________________________.

   e. ______________________________.

4. List three inhalant allergens given in this lesson to which a person could be allergic.

   a. ______________________________.

   b. ______________________________.

   c. ______________________________.

5. List four food allergens mentioned in the lesson that might cause an asthma attack.

   a. ____.

   b. ____.

   c. ____.

   d. ____.

6. List three irritant inhalants mentioned in the lesson.

   a. ____.

   b. ____.

   c. ____.

7. ________________________________ asthma is more common among adults over 35, especially women.

8. List four signs/symptoms of triad asthma.

   a. ____.

   b. ____.

   c. ____.

   d. ____.

9. Wheezing in a particular part of the body indicates __________________________

   ____

10. List two reasons for hospitalizing a patient with asthma.

    a. ______________________________________.

    b. ______________________________________.

11. The purpose of long term asthma therapy is ______________________________

    ____

12. Which response is **NOT** part of the treatment for an adult having an acute asthma/attack?

    a. Open the airway.

    b. Give humidifier oxygen or a nebulizer.

    c. Give a sedative to relax the patient.

    d. Establish an IV with D5W or D5 normal saline.

    e. Use a bronchodilator such as epinephrine.

Check Your Answers on Next Page

SOLUTIONS TO EXERCISES, LESSON 4

1. Chronic obstructive pulmonary diseases. (para 4-1a)

2. These passageways to close partially. (para 4-1a)

3. Extrinsic (allergic)asthma.
   Intrinsic asthma.
   Triad asthma.
   Nasal polyp asthma.
   Bronchospasm. (para 4-1c)

4. You are correct if your listed any three of the following:

   Pollens.
   Dusts.
   Animal danders.
   Feathers.
   Molds. (para 4-2a(1))

5. You are correct if you listed any four of the following:

   Milk.
   Eggs.
   Nuts.
   Chocolate.
   Fish.
   Shellfish.
   Strawberries. (para 4-2a(2))

6. Fumes.
   Cold air.
   Air pollutants. (para 4-2a(3))

7. Intrinsic. (para 4-2b)

8. You are correct if you listed any four of the following:

Respiratory distress.
Cough.
Floushing.
Cyanosis.
Apprehension.
Tachycardia.
Perspiration.
Flaring of nasal alae.
Dyspnea.
Patient sitting up.
Wheezing. (paras 4-2c(1)(a)-(j))

9. An obstruction by a foreign body or a tumor in the area. (para 4-2c(2)(e))

10. You are correct if you listed any two of the following:

Seventy-two hours of unremitting asthma.
One hour of adequate acute therapy without improvement.
Three trips to the emergency room in three days.
Quiet chest.
Pulse rate which varies more than 10mm Hg.
Sternocleidomastoid muscle and intercostal muscle withdrawing.
Low carbon dioxide pressure (PCO_2). (paras 4-4b(1)-(7))

11. To identify the cause of and prevent asthma attacks. (para 4-4d)

12. c. (paras 4-4f(1)(a)-(f))

End of Lesson 4

LESSON ASSIGNMENT

LESSON 5 Respiratory Disorders.

TEXT ASSIGNMENT Paragraphs 5-1 through 5-17.

LESSON OBJECTIVES After completing this lesson, you should be able to:

5-1. Identify the characteristics, signs/symptoms, and treatment for hyperventilation syndrome.

5-2. Identify the characteristics, signs/symptoms, and treatment for spontaneous pneumothorax.

5-3. Identify the characteristics, signs/symptoms, and treatment for pulmonary embolism.

5-4. Identify the characteristics, signs/symptoms, and treatment for inhaled toxic substances.

SUGGESTION After completing the assignment, complete the exercises at the end of this lesson. These exercises will help you to achieve the lesson objectives.

LESSON 5

RESPIRATORY DISORDERS

Section I. HYPERVENTILATION SYNDROME

5-1. DEFINITION/CHARACTERISTICS

a. **Hyperventilation.** Hyperventilation, a common response to phsychological stress, is a condition that develops as a result of an individual breathing too deeply and too rapidly. Blood pH (hydrogen ion) is raised above normal, and the body experiences alkalosis (a condition in which the blood pH is between 7.45 and 8.00). By breathing as rapidly as possible for three to five minutes, a person can bring on the signs and symptoms of hyperventilation deliberately.

b. **Hyperventilation Syndrome.** Patients who are anxious and often feel fatigue, nervousness, and dizziness may suffer from hyperventilation syndrome. The individual may breathe rapidly, breathing out so much carbon dioxide that he becomes unconscious. Unconscious, he begins to breath normally again, the carbon dioxide level becomes normal, and he regains consciousness. When the patient becomes nervous and anxious again, he is likely to experience hyperventilation syndrome again.

5-2. SIGNS/SYMPTOMS

The following signs/symptoms are characteristic of a hyperventilation syndrome attack:

a. Nervousness.

b. Tachypnea--rate of breathing is excessively high (for adults over 25 respirations/per minute).

c. "Unable to catch breath."

d. Dizziness.

e. Tingling or numbness around mouth or in hands and feet.

f. Carpopedal spasm--spasm of muscles in the carpus (the joint between the hand and the wrist and/or spasm of muscles in the foot).

5-3. TREATMENT

Calm the patient and have him breathe into a paper bag. This will cause the patient to breathe his own exhaled breath (which is high in carbon dioxide). In that process, the patient will raise the carbon dioxide level in his body.

Section II. SPONTANEOUS PNEUMOTHORAX

5-4. DEFINITION/CHARACTERICS

a. In spontaneous pneumothorax, a weak area in the surface of the lungs will rupture for no apparent reason, allowing air to leak into the chest cavity. The affected lung collapses and loses its ability to expand normally. There are all degrees of this condition, from the patient who is not particularly uncomfortable to the patient who suffers respiratory distress and must be taken to the hospital.

b. Other causes of pneumothorax include the following:

(1) Perforation of the pleura by erosion through the diaphragm.

(2) During the course of a pulmonary disease such as tuberculosis, an abcess, or emphysema.

(3) Rupture of a bleb (a large weak vessel).

(4) Coughing.

(5) Exertion.

(6) Rapid altitude changes; for example, a parachute drop.

(7) Diving.

5-5. SIGNS/SYMPTOMS

Signs and symptoms include the following:

a. Dry, hacking cough.

b. Sudden sharp chest pain or vague chest discomfort.

c. Dyspnea (labored or difficult breathing).

d. Pain in shoulder and arm.

e. In tension pneumothorax, the percussion note is hyperresonant (louder) over the involved side.

f. Diminished motion on the affected side.

5-6. DIAGNOSIS

A chest x-ray may be used to confirm the diagnosis of pneumothorax. A film taken when the patient exhales will show air in the pleural space with a visible border of retracted lung. The lung may have retracted in one area only.

5-7. TREATMENT

a. **Small Pneumothorax.** No special treatment is required as the air is reabsorbed in a few days.

b. **Bilateral Pneumothorax.** Introduce a chest tube with water- sealed drainage. Suction the air out of the chest cavity so that the lung can expand rapidly.

c. **Tension Pneumothorax.** Insert a short, beveled needle or a chest tube into the front part of the affected area of the chest and drain the air or fluid from the chest cavity.

Section III. PULMONARY EMBOLISM

5-8. DEFINITION/CHARACTERISTICS

Pulmonary embolism is defined as the sudden blocking of a pulmonary artery or one of its branches by a blood clot or other obstruction. The obstruction is carried to the site by the blood current. For example, blood clots may form in the veins of the legs or pelvis and be carried through the veins, through the right heart, where they reach the narrowing network of pulmonary vessels. Factors that favor the development of such obstructions include the following:

a. **Prolonged Immobilization.** Blood becomes stagnant in the lower extremities of bedridden patients, and blood clots can form. A lower extremity in a cast is also conducive to blood clot formation.

b. **Thrombophlebitis (Inflammation of the Veins).** A patient suffering from thrombophlebitis in the pelvis or legs may have blood clots form in either of those area.

c. **Drugs.** An individual taking certain drugs--for example, birth control pills--has a higher risk of developing blood clots.

d. **Fat Particles.** Other substances in addition to blood clots may cause an obstruction in an artery. Particles of fat may break loose during a severe injury to the body, be carried by the bloodstream, and lodge in an artery.

e. **Amniotic Fluid.** During childbirth, amniotic fluid may enter the mother's circulatory system and move into the mother's lungs.

5-9. SIGNS/SYMPTOMS

The signs and symptoms of pulmonary embolism vary with the size of the obstruction. The typical patient may have a sudden onset of severe, unexplained dyspnea (sharp chest pain made worse by coughing or deep breathing), tachycardia (rapid heart rate, over 100 beats per minute), labored breathing, and falling blood pressure. A chest examination may show no abnormalities, however.

5-10. DIAGNOSIS/PHYSICAL EXAMINATION

a. **Perform an Auscultation Examination.** Listen for atelectatic rales (fine, rattling sounds in a lung which is not completely expanded). Also, listen for localized wheezes (high-pitched notes like musical sounds).

b. **Take the Pulse.** The pulse rate may be over 100 beats per minute (tachycardia).

NOTE: A deep tenderness in the calf area of the leg may indicate phlebitis.

5-11. TREATMENT

a. **In the Field.** Treatment is largely supportive since definitive therapy with anticoagulants requires hospitalization. Follow this procedure:

(1) Ensure an open airway.

(2) Assist ventilations as needed.

(3) Administer oxygen in the highest possible concentration.

(4) Establish an IV lifeline with a solution of water with five percent dextrose (D5W) and monitor the patient's cardiac rhythm.

b. **In the Hospital.** Treatment in the hospital includes these procedures:

(1) Bed rest.

(2) Analgesics to relieve pain, perhaps a narcotic.

(3) Oxygen.

(4) Intravenous (IV) therapy.

(5) Treatment for shock, if present.

(6) Warm packs for thrombophlebitis (inflammation of a vein).

(7) Anticoagulation medication such as heparin or Coumadin.

(8) Surgical ligation (tying or binding the vein) or embolectomy (surgical removal of the blood clot).

5-12. PREVENTION OF VENOUS STASIS

Increased pressure on veins causes the veins to become abnormally dilated; this condition is referred to as venous stasis. Such veins are most commonly seen in the superficial veins of the legs. Elastic hose and leg exercises help prevent venous stasis. In severe cases, amputation may be necessary.

Section IV. INHALED TOXIC SUBSTANCES

5-13. DEFINITION/CHARACTERISTICS

Inhaled toxic substances refer to combustion and chemical irritants that a person breathes in, thus damaging parts of his body. Damage may be caused by such things as a blast of hot, wet air (steam), or poisonous gas. The damage done to the body may be obstruction due to edema in the airway and alveoli, a bronchospasm attack, or chemical pulmonary edema.

5-14. TOXIC AGENTS (INHALANTS)

Gases that combine with water to form corrosive acids or alkali fumes that cause burns to the upper respiratory tract are toxic agents. Other toxic agents include:

a. Ammonia - ammonium hydroxide.

b. Nitrogen oxide - nitric oxide.

c. Sulfur dioxide - sulfurous acid.

d. Decomposed chlorinated hydrocarbons.

e. Chlorine gas - found in swimming pools.

5-15. PATIENT HISTORY/PHYSICAL EXAMINATION

a. **Patient History**. When taking patient history, be sure to include this specific information:

(1) The duration of exposure to the toxic inhalant.

(2) Whether the patient was in a closed or open environment during exposure. If the patient was in a closed environment, he is more liable to have respiratory tract damage. Inhaling of a substance in the open, however, can cause similar damage to the respiratory tract.

(3) Whether the patient lost consciousness. If the patient lost consciousness, mechanisms that usually protect the lower respiratory tract may not have functioned.

(4) Identity of the toxic agent(s), if possible.

b. **Physical Examination**. The physical examination of the patient suffering from inhalation of toxic substances should include inspection of the mouth and face, visual examination of the throat, and auscultation of the chest.

5-16. COMMON SIGNS/SYMPTOMS

A person who has inhaled something toxic will commonly experience irritation to the eyes, sneezing, coughing, dyspnea (labored or difficult breathing), and/or choking.

5-17. TREATMENT

a. First, establish and maintain an airway.

CAUTION: If laryngeal edema develops rapidly, you may need to perform an endotracheal intubation or cricothyrotomy in the field.

b. Assist ventilation as needed.

c. Administer humidified oxygen in the highest concentration available to all toxic inhalant patients, whether they seem to need oxygen or not.

d. Establish an IV lifeline with a solution of water with five percent dextrose.

e. Monitor cardiac rhythm and general status of patients who have suffered intense exposure to smoke or toxic fumes. Continue monitoring for 18 to 24 hours.

f. Refer to Table 5-1, Toxic Inhalants, for signs/symptoms and treatments for ammonia gas, nitrogen oxide, sulfur oxide (SMDG), and cholorinated hydrocarbons-petroleum distillates.

SIGNS/SYMPTOMS	TREATMENT
A. Ammonia gas	
1. Irritation of eyes and respiratory tract. 2. Cough. 3. Choking. 4. Abdominal pain.	1. Flush eyes with tap water for 15 minutes. 2. Give severe positive pressure oxygen to prevent pulmonary edema. 3. Support respirations.
B. Nitrogen Oxide	
1. Local burning in eyes, nasal pharyngeal, or mucous membranes. 2. Fatigue. 3. Cough. 4. Dyspnea. 5. Pulmonary edema. 6. Later, bronchitis, pneumonia.	1. Absolute bed rest. 2. Pure oxygen as soon as symptoms develop. 3. For excessive pulmonary foam, suction. 4. Postural drainage.
C. Sulfur Oxide (SMDG)	
1. Respiratory tract irritation. 2. Sneezing. 3. Cough. 4. Dyspnea. 5. Pulmonary edema.	1. Remove from contaminated area. 2. Give oxygen positive pressure breathing. 3. Respiratory support.
D. Chlorinated Hydrocarbons--Petroleum Distillates	
1. Euphoria. 2. Burning in chest. 3. Headache. 4. Weakness. 5. CNS depression. 6. Confusion.	1. Oxygen. 2. Support respirations.

Table 5-1. Toxic inhalants.

Continue with Exercises

EXERCISES, LESSON 5

INSTRUCTIONS. Answer these exercises by writing the answer in the space provided. After you have answered all the exercises, turn to "Solutions to Exercises" at the end of the lesson and check your answers.

1. An individual who breathes too deeply and too rapidly can bring on a condition called ______________________________________.

2. Sometimes a weak area in the surface of the lungs will rupture allowing air to leak into the chest cavity; the resulting condition is called __________________.

3. A chest x-ray showing air in the pleural space with a visible border of retracted lung when the patient exhales is an indication that he suffers from ____________.

4. List three causes of pulmonary embolism.

   a. ____.

   b. ____.

   c. ____.

5. A person having a deep tenderness in the calf area of the leg may be suffering from ____.

6. List three signs/symptoms of hyperventilation.

   a. ____.

   b. ____.

   c. ____.

7. A person suffering from __________________ should breathe into a paper bag.

8. List three types of spontaneous pneumothorax are:

   a. ____.

   b. ____.

   c. ____.

9. The patient has inhaled a toxic substance. List four items of information that should be included when taking this patient's history.

   a. ____.

   b. ____.

   c. ____.

   d. ____.

Check Your Answers on Next Page

SOLUTIONS TO EXERCISES, LESSON 5

1. Hyperventilation. (para 5-1a)

2. Spontaneous pneumothorax. (para 5-4a)

3. Pneumothorax. (para 5-6)

4. You are correct if you listed any three of the following:

    Prolonged immobilization.
    Inflammation of the veins.
    Drugs.
    Fat particles.
    Amniotic fluid. (para 5-8a through e)

5. Plebitis. (para 5-10c)

6. You are correct if you listed any three of the following:

    Nervousness.
    Tachypnea.
    Unable to catch breath.
    Dizziness.
    Tingling or numbness around mouth or in hands and feet.
    Carpopedal spasm. (para 5-2a-f)

7. Hyperventilation. (para 5-3)

8. Small pneumothorax.
   Bilateral pneumothorax.
   Tension pneumothorax. (paras 5-7a, b, c)

9. Duration of exposure to toxic agents.
   Whether the patient was in an open or closed environment.
   Whether the patient lost consciousness.
   Identity of toxic agents. (paras 5-15a(1)-(4))

End of Lesson 5

LESSON ASSIGNMENT

LESSON 6 Tuberculosis.

TEXT ASSIGNMENT Paragraphs 6-1 through 6-11.

LESSON OBJECTIVES After completing this lesson, you should be able to:

6-1. Identify the characteristics, signs/ symptoms, diagnosis, and treatment for tuberculosis.

6-2. Identify the reservoir, sources, and transmission of tuberculosis infection.

6-3. Identify the measures in the tuberculosis control program.

SUGGESTION After completing the assignment, complete the exercises at the end of this lesson. These exercises will help you to achieve the lesson objectives.

LESSON 6

TUBERCULOSIS

6-1. DEFINITION

Tuberculosis is a chronic disease caused by the bacteria Mycobacterium tuberculosis. The initial disease may not be noticed, but eventually the infection may spread to various parts of the body--tuberculosis of the bones and joints; intestinal tuberculosis; urinary tract tuberculosis. The incidence of tuberculosis is less today than in the past. In the United States Army in World War II, the number of tuberculosis cases was 1 per 1,000 soldiers. By 1982, only 250,000 cases were reported in the United States. The decline in the number of cases can be attributed to three factors: education about causes of tuberculosis; better diet and nutritional information; and early diagnosis and treatment of tuberculosis cases.

6-2. COMMUNICABILITY OF INFECTION

a. **Reservoir, Sources, Transmission Route.** The most common reservoir of tuberculosis is man, and the source of infection is respiratory secretion of individuals who have active pulmonary lesions. Tuberculous bacteria may be transmitted by direct or indirect contact with the patient who has open lesions. The most common route of transmission, however, is by inhaling airborne droplet nuclei. When a patient coughs or sneezes, a person may inhale the bacteria in the air and, if susceptible, may contract tuberculosis. Family, military, and institutional living can contribute to the spread of tuberculosis if a person has an active case that is unrecognized and, consequently, untreated. A reservoir for Mycobacterium bovis, the bovine strain of tuberculosis, is diseased cattle. Man ingests this bacillus by drinking the raw milk from such cattle. Man may also contract this type of tuberculosis by inhaling airborne organisms in and around barns that have infected animals or by handling infectious animal products. Since herds of animals are continuously tested for tuberculosis and milk is pasteurized, this form of tuberculosis has been controlled.

b. **Incubation Period.** The incubation period is usually about four to six weeks from the time of effective exposure to the appearance of a primary lesion of first infection. The time between the first infection and reinfection of tuberculosis may be many years. If the individual is reinfected, the length of time necessary for new lesions to develop depends on the general health of the person and the source and numbers of organisms entering his system.

c. **Communicability.** A patient is infectious for as long as he discharges tubercle bacilli. The degree of communicability depends on several factors: density of contaminated droplets in the air; coughing habits of the patient; and air circulation and fallout in the particular environment. During the period when the patient is infectious, an uninfected person needs to inhale at least one infectious droplet nucleus to become infected. The healthy person must inhale tubercle bacilli so that they are carried far down the airways to a point in the lung where fixed mononuclear phagocytes can pick the droplets up and droplet intracellular multiplication can begin. The infected patient's sputum, if it carries enough bacilli, is a source of infection when the patient coughs or sneezes thus spraying the air with bacilli. If there are several people living close together, just one of them being infected with tuberculous bacilli can spread the disease to the others.

d. **Immunity.** How susceptible people are to infection in general is influenced by several factors: age, sex, race, nutrition, and general health. In regard to tuberculosis, children under 3 years old are the most susceptible. There have been fewer cases of tuberculosis in children since bovine tuberculosis has been controlled. (Children are no longer consuming infected dairy products.) There are fewer cases of tuberculosis among Caucasians than among Blacks and American Indians, but no one is sure of the reason. Perhaps through the years only Caucasians most resistant to tuberculosis have survived. In general, possibly Caucasians live in better environments and eat more nutritionally balanced meals thus giving them better health. The number of cases of tuberculosis is usually greater among city dwellers than among those who live in the country. City people live closer together; therefore, one infected city dweller will probably come in contact with and pass on the tuberculosis infection to more people than a country dweller.

6-3. SIGNS/SYMPTOMS

From the time of infection, it takes about four to eight weeks for a person to develop tuberculosis. The person may have no symptoms, mild symptoms, or nonspecific symptoms. If there are symptoms, these are the most common:

a. Fatigue.

b. Anorexia.

c. Weight loss.

d. Irregular menses.

e. Low grade fever.

f. Night sweats.

g. Cough (which has no specific characteristics).

h. Hemoptysis (blood in the sputum).

i. Pleuritic chest pain (pain in the pleural chest cavity).

6-4. TYPES OF TESTS

a. **Chest X-ray**. In almost all cases, a chest x-ray will show the disease. A single chest x-ray is not usually enough to diagnose tuberculosis. This is because tuberculosis lesions behind ribs, cardiovascular structures, and the diaphragm will not show up on a chest x-ray for tuberculosis. Several chest x-rays, therefore, are needed to establish the activity of the bacilli and to select and determine the appropriate treatment.

b. **Tuberculin Skin Testing**. The basis of tuberculin skin tests is that the skin is hypersensitive to a specific bacterial protein antigen. Administer the antigen and examine the induration (hardening of the area on which the antigen was placed). A positive reaction (induration 10 mm or more in diameter) indicates only exposure to tuberculosis; it does not necessarily mean that the person has tuberculosis. To find out whether the person has tuberculosis now, use x-ray or bacteriological methods. People who have a negative tuberculin reaction include the following: those who have never been infected; those who are in the preallergic early stage of first infection, and, strangely enough, those with advanced terminal tuberculosis.

(1) Tine test. The tine test uses dried, old tuberculin (OT) on multiple metal tines (sharp, pointed prongs like a fork) which are in a round, plastic head. When the tines are pressed against an individual's skin, the antigen is forced between layers of the skin in the same manner as an injection. This method of testing is safe and convenient for mass surveys. The site where the test was done should be read between 48 and 72 hours after the test was performed. What the site looks like determines whether the test resulted in a positive take, a doubtful take, or a negative take as noted below:

(a) Positive take -- induration but no erythema (abnormal) skin redness.

(b) Doubtful take -- 2 mm induration.

(c) Negative take -- less than 2 mm induration.

(2) Mantoux test. This test, used for adult testing, must be used if the tine test is doubtful or positive. The test requires intradermal injection of antigen 0.1 ml (1 I.U.) of purified protein derivative (PPD). If a fairly high level of susceptibility is expected, 0.1 ml (0.5 I.U.) of PPD may be used. Read from 48 to 72 hours. Note the following information:

(a) Positive take -- 10 mm induration or more.

(b) Doubtful take -- 5 mm through 9 mm induration.

(c) Negative take -- less than 5 mm induration.

(3) Conversion. Conversion refers to a positive reaction that has occurred within one year after a known negative reaction. If the person tested is under 35 years old, begin treatment for tuberculosis immediately.

6-5. GENERAL CARE

How rapidly and/or how well tuberculosis lesions heal depends on two factors: specific drug treatment and the body's defense mechanism. Bed rest is necessary only if the patient has a fever, hemoptysis (blood-stained sputum), or a severe cough. A patient with any of these symptoms may need a few weeks of bed rest. The patient whose sputum contains tuberculosis bacilli should be isolated until effective treatment has been given for at least two weeks. Generally, these and other patients whose drug treatment has been established can return to normal physical activity.

6-6. DRUG THERAPY

Drug treatment must continue for at least eighteen to twenty-four months. A minimum of two drugs should be used concurrently, but there is a strong trend toward the use of three drugs. Drug therapy appears to be most effective when taken in a simple daily dose on an empty stomach.

a. **Isoniazid (INH).**

(1) Drug use. This drug should always be included in the original treatment and always used in conjunction with other anti-tuberculosis drugs. The dosage for adults is 5 mg/kg per day up to 300 mg per day. This is the most effective drug at the present time; however, there may be adverse reactions.

(2) Adverse reactions. If the dosage is the usual 5 mg/kg daily, adverse reactions to isoniazid are unusual. Cases of hepatitis thought to have been caused by the drug have been reported. If the patient has a liver dysfunction, be cautious in prescribing the drug. Tell patients to be sure to stop taking the drug and notify the doctor if any adverse signs/symptoms occur. A patient taking large doses of isoniazid may experience peripheral neuropathy (disturbances in the peripheral nervous system) and, occasionally, central nervous system irritability caused by depletion of pyridoxine, one of the forms of vitamin B6. Urine retention is another possible adverse reaction from isoniazid.

b. **Rifampin (Rifadin®).** This drug, a semisynthetic derivative of rifamycin, is given orally and usually well tolerated. The drug distributes readily into all body tissue fluids including the cerebral spinal fluid (CSF). The dosage is 600 mg (2--300 mg caps). Rifampin must be used along with another anti-tuberculosis drug. Adverse reactions include anorexia, diarrhea, and headache.

c. **Streptomycin.**

(1) Drug use. Streptomycin, less effective than isoniazid in advanced tuberculosis cases, must be given in conjunction with other drugs. The dosage is 1-2 mg daily by intramuscular injection.

(2) Adverse reactions. If streptomycin is used daily, the drug may cause eighth nerve damage (vertigo, deafness). If the drug is continued, the damage may be irreversible. Occasionally, the patient suffers generalized dermatitis (inflammation of the skin) in which case use of the drug must be discontinued.

d. **Ethambutol (Myambutol®).**

(1) Drug use. Ethambutol, the principal second line drug, must be used in combination with another drug, normally isoniazid. Ethambutol will prevent the development of organisms which are resistant to major drugs. The dosage is 15 mg/kg, given orally.

(2) Adverse effects. This drug has few side effects. Optic neuritis (inflammation of the optic nerve) is one possible side effect, but it is usually minor and reversible. Before and during treatment with this drug, the patient's clarity of vision should be checked. If vision becomes less clear, the use of this drug should be discontinued. Since clearness of vision cannot be properly checked in infants and young children, avoid using ethambutol with these patients.

e. **Bacille Calmette-Guerin (BCG) Vaccine.** This vaccine, administered intradermally, is a living, attenuated strain of tubercle bacilli of bovine origin. The vaccine offers no positive protection to tuberculin-negative people but can give false-positive readings. The vaccine converts at least 90 percent of tuberculin-negative people to a state of skin sensitivity. The protection given by vaccination is only partial, and no one is quite sure how long the vaccination lasts. Mass vaccination with this vaccine is applicable only in situations where risk of infection and the number of tuberculin-negative contacts of active disease are both high.

(1) Drug use. The dosage is 50 mg per day by mouth. Use pyridoxine (B6) only if the patient experiences side effects when taking isoniazid. This drug is not used routinely.

(2) Adverse effects. Adverse effects include irritability or depression.

6-7. VACCINATION SITE REACTION

Read the vaccination site this way. A skin induration of 10 mm or more is considered a reaction. Less than 10 mm induration is a nonreaction. Read the vaccination site using a millimeter ruler and only the amount of induration, not the skin redness. Reactions are classified in these three types: a positive reaction; a negative reaction; and a conversion reaction.

6-8. POSITIVE REACTION

The induration is 10 mm or more in diameter and indicates that the person has a tuberculin infection now or has had an infection in the past. Two to eights weeks after a person is infected with the tubercule bacillus, the skin test may provide a positive reaction. Disadvantaged people in all countries have a higher rate of positive reactions.

6-9. NEGATIVE REACTION

Induration less than 5 mm in diameter is considered a negative reaction and indicates that a tuberculosis infection is unlikely. A variety of factors make it possible for the tuberculin reaction to decrease in size or even disappear even though the person has tuberculosis. These factors include overwhelming tuberculosis, exanthematous (eruptive) diseases, corticosteroid treatment, sarcoidosis, debility, and increased age. Also consider that there may be something wrong with the materials used in testing. If you suspect that the person may have tuberculosis, even though the reaction is negative, give that test again or use another method of testing for tuberculosis.

6-10. CONVERSION REACTION

A positive reaction that has developed within a year after a negative reaction is called a conversion reaction. This means that the skin induration has changed from a skin induration of less than 10 mm in diameter a year ago to a skin induration greater than 10 mm in diameter and that the increase in the size of the induration is at least 6 mm. The importance of this finding is that it indicates that the person may have had a tuberculosis infection recently. That person will need to be checked periodically because the possibility of developing tuberculosis is greatest during the first two years after an infection.

6-11. GENERAL MEASURE OF CONTROL

It is more difficult to control outbreaks of respiratory infections (including tuberculosis) than many other types of communicable diseases. In general, control efforts are based on improving personal hygiene, avoiding contacts with patients and carriers, controlling dust and aerial contamination, preventing overcrowding and fatigue, and immunizing when applicable.

a. **Avoidance of Direct Contact**. Patients with a respiratory disease such as tuberculosis must be diagnosed, isolated if necessary, and treated as soon as possible. Additionally, these patients should learn and practice personal hygiene measures such as covering the mouth when coughing or sneezing.

b. **Person Hygiene**. Personal hygiene is one of the most important respiratory disease control measures. The approach is through the practice of simple health habits. Covering the nose and mouth when sneezing or coughing and washing the hands should be routine practices. People infected should avoid contact with healthy persons. Personal articles such as towels, drinking glasses, and toothbrushes are not shared. Healthful exercise, fresh air, and sunshine should be encouraged.

Continue with Exercises

EXERCISES, LESSON 6

INSTRUCTIONS. Answer these exercises by writing the answer in the space provided. After you have answered all the exercises, turn to "Solutions to Exercises" at the end of the lesson and check your answers.

1. Tuberculosis, a chronic disease, is caused by ______________________.

2. List three reasons for the decline in the number of tuberculosis cases.

   a. ______________________________________.

   b. ______________________________________.

   c. ______________________________________.

3. List four signs/symptoms of tuberculosis.

   a. ______________________________________.

   b. ______________________________________.

   c. ______________________________________.

   d. ______________________________________.

4. Two methods of diagnosis for tuberculosis are ____________________ and tuberculin skin testing.

5. List two methods of transmission of tuberculosis.

   a. ______________________________________.

   b. ______________________________________.

6. Two types of skin tests which can be used to diagnose tuberculosis are the _________________ test and the _______________________ test.

7. Both types of skin tests are based on the fact that ______________________.

8. List three adverse reactions that isoniazid, the drug of choice in tuberculosis treatment, can have.

   a. ____.

   b. ____.

   c. ____.

9. A tuberculosis treatment drug that moves readily into all the body tissue fluids, including the cerebral spinal fluid, is ________________________________.

10. Vertigo and generalized dermatitis are adverse reactions a patient may experience if being treated for tuberculosis with the drug _________________.

11. Name an adverse reaction which might be experienced by a patient taking the drug ethambutol for tuberculosis ________________________________.

12. _________________________ vaccine is recommended only for individuals working in areas with high exposure to tuberculosis.

13. A tuberculosis patient can infect others as long as the patient discharges ___________________________________.

14. List three reasons when a tuberculosis patient would need bed rest.

    a. ____.

    b. ____.

    c. ____..

15. The length of time between exposure to tuberculosis and the appearance of a primary lesion of first infection is usually about ___________________________.

Check Your Answers on Next Page

SOLUTIONS TO EXERCISES, LESSON 6

1. The bacteria Mycobacterium tuberculosis. (para 6-1)

2. You are correct if you listed any three of the following:

   Education.
   Diet.
   Preventive measures.
   Early diagnosis. (para 6-1)

3. You are correct if you listed any four of the following:

   Fatigue.
   Anorexia.
   Weight Loss.
   Irregular menses.
   Night sweats.
   Cough.
   Blood-stained sputum.
   Pleuritic chest pain.
   Low grade fever. (paras 6-3a-i)

4. Chest x-ray. (para 6-4a)

5. Inhaling an airborne droplet which has the tuberculosis bacteria.
   Drinking raw milk from cattle infected with the bovine strain of tuberculosis. (para 6-2)

6. Tine; Mantoux. (paras 6-4b(1),(2))

7. The skin is hypersensitive to a specific bacterial protein antigen. (para 6-4b)

8. You are correct if you listed any three of the following:

   Peripheral neuropathy.
   Central nervous system irritability.
   Urine retention.
   Depletion of vitamin B6. (para 6-6a(2))

9. Rifampin also called Rifadin[R]. (para 6-6b)

10. Streptomycin. (para 6-6c(2)

11. Optic neuritis. (para 6-6d(2)(b)

12. Bacille Calmette-Guerin (BCG). (para 6-6e)

13. Tubercle bacille. (para 6-2c)

14. Patient has a fever.
    Patient has blood-stained sputum.
    Patient has severe cough. (para 6-5)

15. Four to six weeks. (para 6-2b)

End of Lesson 6

This page intentionally left blank.

Chest and Airway Problems

Subcourse MD0569

This page intentionally left blank.

U.S. ARMY MEDICAL DEPARTMENT CENTER AND SCHOOL
FORT SAM HOUSTON, TEXAS 78234-6100

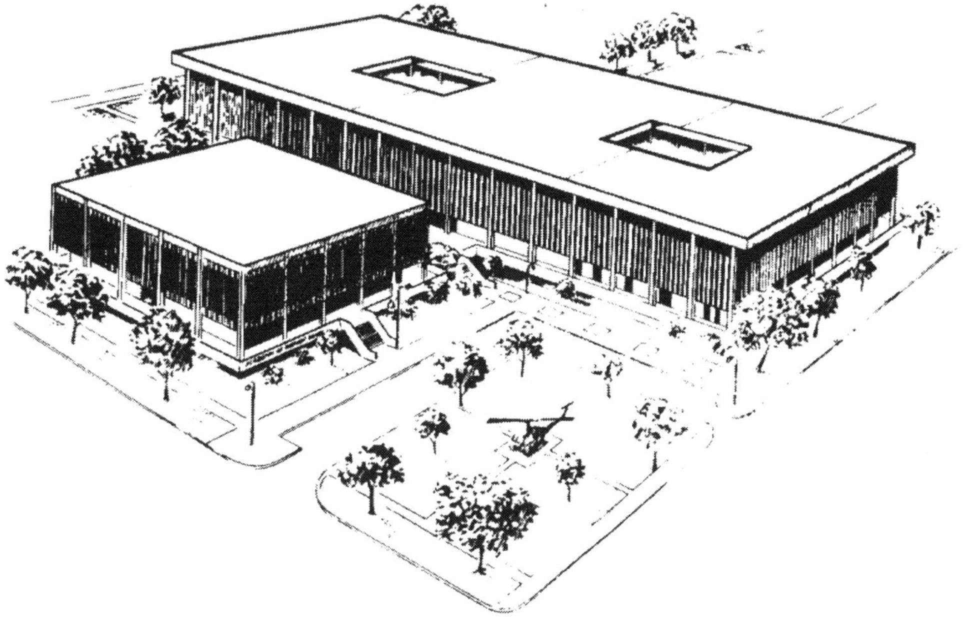

CHEST AND AIRWAY PROBLEMS

SUBCOURSE MD0569 EDITION 100

DEVELOPMENT

This subcourse is approved for resident and correspondence course instruction. It reflects the current thought of the Academy of Health Sciences and conforms to printed Department of the Army doctrine as closely as currently possible. Development and progress render such doctrine continuously subject to change.

The subject matter expert responsible for content accuracy of this edition was the NCOIC, Nursing Science Division, DSN 471-3086 or area code (210) 221-3086, M6 Branch, Academy of Health Sciences, ATTN: MCCS-HNP, Fort Sam Houston, Texas 78234-6100.

ADMINISTRATION

Students who desire credit hours for this correspondence subcourse must meet eligibility requirements and must enroll in the subcourse. Application for enrollment should be made at the Internet website: http://www.atrrs.army.mil. You can access the course catalog in the upper right corner. Enter School Code 555 for medical correspondence courses. Copy down the course number and title. To apply for enrollment, return to the main ATRRS screen and scroll down the right side for ATRRS Channels. Click on SELF DEVELOPMENT to open the application and then follow the on screen instructions.

For comments or questions regarding enrollment, student records, or examination shipments, contact the Nonresident Instruction Branch at DSN 471-5877, commercial (210) 221-5877, toll-free 1-800-344-2380; fax: 210-221-4012 or DSN 471-4012, e-mail accp@amedd.army.mil, or write to:

NONRESIDENT INSTRUCTION BRANCH
AMEDDC&S
ATTN: MCCS-HSN
2105 11TH STREET SUITE 4191
FORT SAM HOUSTON TX 78234-5064

CLARIFICATION OF TERMINOLOGY

When used in this publication, words such as "he," "him," "his," and "men" 'are intended to include both the masculine and feminine genders, unless specifically stated otherwise or when obvious in context.

TABLE OF CONTENTS

Lesson | **Paragraphs**

INTRODUCTION

1 CHEST TRAUMA

Section I General Information About Chest injuries. 1-1--1-5
Section II Specific Chest Injuries 1-6--1-13
Section III Chest Decompression 1-14--1-16
Exercises

2 AIRWAY MANAGEMENT

Section I Esophageal Obturator Airway 2-1--2-6
Section II Endotracheal Tube 2-7--2-13
Exercises

3 CRICOTHYROIDOTOMY

Section I General Considerations 3-1--3-4
Section II Needle Cricothyroidotomy 3-5--3-6
Section III Surgical Cricothyroidotomy 3-7--3-9
Exercises

CORRESPONDENCE COURSE OF
THE U.S. ARMY MEDICAL DEPARTMENT CENTER AND SCHOOL

SUBCOURSE MD0569

CHEST AND AIRWAY PROBLEMS

INTRODUCTION

In this subcourse, you will study chest and airway problems. Chest trauma refers to general information about chest injuries as well as information about specific chest injuries. Airway problems includes information on devices--the esophageal obturator airway (EOA), the esophageal gastric tube airway (EGTA), and the endotracheal tube (ET)--that can be used to open and maintain an airway. If other life-saving methods are not successful in opening and maintaining an airway, an opening is made in the trachea to bypass the site of an upper airway obstruction. This subject matter is of vital importance in saving lives.

<u>Subcourse Components</u>:

The subcourse instructional material consists of four lessons as follows:

Lesson 1, Chest Trauma.
Lesson 2, Airway Management.
Lesson 3, Cricothyroidotomy.

Here are some suggestions that may be helpful to you in completing this subcourse:

--Read and study each lesson carefully.

--Complete the subcourse lesson by lesson. After completing each lesson, work the exercises at the end of the lesson, marking your answers in this booklet.

--After completing each set of lesson exercises, compare your answers with those on the solution sheet that follows the exercises. If you have answered an exercise incorrectly, check the reference cited after the answer on the solution sheet to determine why your response was not the correct one.

Credit Awarded:

Upon successful completion of the examination for this subcourse, you will be awarded 8 credit hours.

To receive credit hours, you must be officially enrolled and complete an examination furnished by the Nonresident Instruction Branch at Fort Sam Houston, Texas.

You can enroll by going to the web site http://atrrs.army.mil and enrolling under "Self Development" (School Code 555).

A listing of correspondence courses and subcourses available through the Nonresident Instruction Section is found in Chapter 4 of DA Pamphlet 350-59, Army Correspondence Course Program Catalog. The DA PAM is available at the following website: http://www.usapa.army.mil/pdffiles/p350-59.pdf.

LESSON ASSIGNMENT

LESSON 1 Chest Trauma

LESSON ASSIGNMENT Paragraphs 1-1 through 1-16.

LESSON OBJECTIVES After completing this lesson, you should be able to:

1-1. Identify common signs, common treatment, and general principles of treatment for chest injuries.

1-2. Define these specific chest injuries and identify the signs/symptoms and treatment of the specific chest injuries:

Fractured ribs or sternum.
Flail chest.
Cardiac contusion.
Hemothorax.
Simple pneumothorax.
Subcutaneous emphysema.
Open pneumothorax.
Tension pneumothorax.

1-3. List the steps in the procedure of two types of chest decompression (needle chest decompression and catheter -over-needle chest decompression) in the order of performance.

SUGGESTION After completing the assignment, complete the exercises of this lesson. These exercises will help you to achieve the lesson objectives.

LESSON 1

CHEST TRAUMA

Section I. GENERAL INFORMATION ABOUT CHEST INJURIES

1-1. INTRODUCTION

Chest injuries are of major importance because they are a common cause of death. Fifty percent of the people who expire from chest injuries die on the way to the hospital. The common causes of penetrating and nonpentrating chest injuries include automobile accidents, falls and blows, gunshot wounds, stab wounds, and crushing injuries. In a chest injury, there is a possibility of internal bleeding and/or direct injury to the heart or lungs; therefore, any chest injury may be serious. Chest decompressions, field functions, and other procedures may be used to save the casualty's life if they are performed correctly and in a timely manner. With specialized training and prescribed methods of treatment for various chest trauma, your ability to recognize and react quickly in each situation is an important factor in regard to whether the casualty survives.

1-2. COMMON SIGNS/SYMPTOMS OF CHEST INJURIES

The common signs and symptoms of chest injuries are:

a. A change in normal breathing pattern.

b. Pain at the site of the injury.

c. Dyspnea (shortness of breath).

d. Failure of the chest to expand.

e. A rapid/weak pulse.

f. Low blood pressure.

g. A dry cough or blood.

h. A sucking sound on respiration.

i. Cyanosis (bluish discoloration of the skin due to lack of oxygen).

j. Hemoptysis (spitting of blood from lesions in the larynx, traches, or lower respiratory tract).

1-3. COMMON TREATMENT FOR CHEST INJURIES

Regardless of the type of chest injury, initial treatment is almost always the same. Begin by examining the casualty to detect the chest injury.

a. Question the casualty, if he is conscious, to see if he has difficulty in breathing.

b. Observe the casualty's bare chest and upper abdomen for respiratory rate and depth.

c. Check for equal movement of both sides of the casualty's chest.

d. Examine the entire chest wall (including the back) beneath any overlying clothing.

e. Listen to the casualty's chest with a stethoscope. Listen to both sides of the chest, comparing both sides for volume, loudness, and equality.

1-4. TYPES OF CHEST INJURIES

a. **Penetrating Injuries.** A penetrating injury may be a hole in the thoracic cavity that allows air inside the thorax, the air filling the thoracic cavity (pneumothorax). A penetrating injury may cause blood to flow into the thoracic cavity (hemothorax), filling the thorax with blood.

b. **Blunt Injuries.** These are blunt injuries: rib and sternum damage; flail chest; and cardiac contusion.

c. **Results of Penetrating/Blunt Injuries**. Penetrating and blunt injuries can cause considerable damage. Both types of injury can cause air to build up outside the lung in the thoracic cavity, and the individual has simple pneumothorax. The pressure has not been great enough to cause the lung to collapse. A blunt injury or a penetrating injury may cause air to build up to such great pressure in the thoracic cavity that the lungs collapse. Tension pneumothorax is the name of this condition.

1-5. GENERAL PRINCIPLES OF TREATMENT FOR CHEST TRAUMA

Follow these general principles in treating for chest trauma:

a. Maintain normal pleural pressure by the use of suction devices throughout the treatment. Keep the pleural space empty by using suctioning devices such as hemovac or pleuralvac. Monitor the suctioning device frequently, regardless of which device is used.

b. Monitor the casualty for pericardial tamponade. This condition, which will be discussed later, is caused by penetrating chest wounds such as gunshot wounds or stab wounds. The result of the condition can be diminished cardiac output and finally death; therefore, it is extremely important to watch for signs of pericardial tamponade in the person.

c. Keep the bronchial tree clear of retained blood, foreign material, and bronchial secretions by using suction as needed.

d. Give oxygen to maintain adequate oxygenation and removal of carbon dioxide. If oxygen administered by nasal catheter is inadequate, use tracheal intubation, cricothyroidotomy, or controlled positive breathing.

e. Estimate the amount of hemorrhage the casualty has, and replace the blood as necessary.

Section II. SPECIFIC CHEST INJURIES

1-6. FRACTURED RIBS OR STERNUM

a. **Fractured Ribs**. Fractured ribs are usually caused by blunt, direct blows or compression injuries of the chest. The upper ribs are protected--in front by the clavicle, in back by the scapulae, in the side by the arms, and by the heavy muscles of the upper thorax and its appendages--and are rarely fractured. The fifth through the ninth ribs are most commonly fractured. The lower two ribs are attached to the thoracic vertebrae and have movement; therefore, they are rarely fractured.

b. **Fractured Sternum**. Fracture of the sternum occurs about once in every twenty chest injuries. Sternum are an indication to look for other serious injuries because a blow hard enough to fracture the sternum will often cause serious damage in the thorax. Injuries associated with a fractured sternum include tracheal or bronchial tears, ruptured diaphragm or esophagus, flail chest, and contusion of the myocardium or lung.

c. **Signs/Symptoms of Fractured Ribs or Sternum.**

(1) Tenderness at the point where the casualty indicates pain.

(2) Pain that worsens when the casualty breathes or coughs.

(3) The casualty may be protecting the affected side by leaning toward that side with his hand protecting it or by splinting the affected side.

(4) Crepitus (grating sounds; sounds which can be heard when bones move against each other).

(5) Subcutaneous emphysema (a condition to be discussed later).

d. **Associated Complications.**

(1) Rupture or lacerations of underlying structures are common. If there is a direct blow to one or more ribs, there is a possibility that the rib ends may be driven into the lung underneath and the pleura, causing damage.

(2) Internal bleeding may be caused by fractured ribs.

(3) Shock.

e. **Treatment.** Treatment includes examining the casualty for underlying chest problems and giving him something for pain.

1-7. FLAIL CHEST

A flail chest occurs when two or more adjacent ribs are fractured in two or more places resulting in a segment of the thoracic cage becoming detached. Flail chest--also called floating or crushed chest--is more common in today's era of high-speed automobile accidents. It is usually caused by a blunt blow to the ribs. If two or more ribs are broken in two places, the part of the chest wall between the breaks collapses and does not participate in the normal expansion of the chest each time the person inhales. When the casualty exhales, the part of the chest wall between the breaks will protrude while the rest of the chest wall contracts.

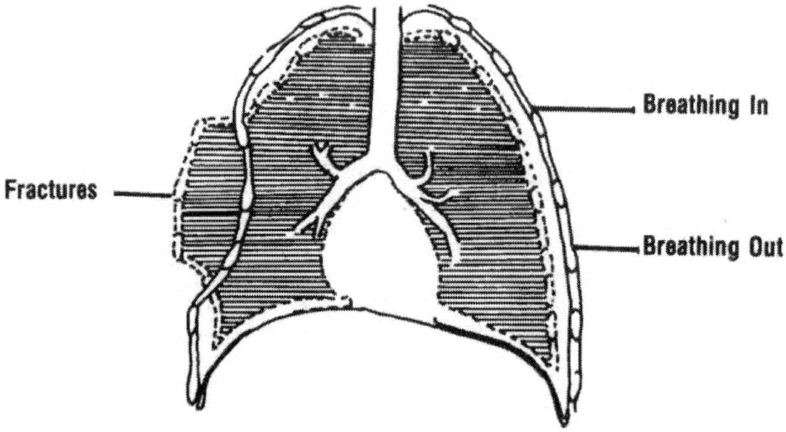

Figure 1-1. Flail chest--paradoxical respirations (active breathing).

a. **Signs/Symptoms.** Signs and symptoms of flail chest include the following:

(1) Pain at the site of the injury.

(2) Tachypnea (rapid breathing).

(3) Paradoxical respirations. For example, the chest expands with expiration (breathing out) and contracts with inhalation (breathing in).

b. **Treatment.** To administer initial treatment to a casualty with a flail chest injury, you should:

(1) Place your hand, a pillow, or another object on the flail segment to immobilize it.

(2) Strap or tape the pillow or other object in place.

(3) Give the casualty oxygen.

1-8. CARDIAC CONTUSION

Cardiac contusion is severe trauma to the anterior chest. This trauma results in bruising and irritation of the heart muscle. This injury is caused by a severe, blunt blow to the chest; for example, a steering wheel injury.

a. **Signs/Symptoms.** Cardiac signs and symptoms include:

(1) Exposed ribs and/or sternum.

(2) Cardiac dysrhythmias may be detectable by an irregular pulse. The location of the injury often influences the types of dysrhythmias. An injury to the right side results in artial dysrhythmias. Injury to the left side or the front results in ventricular dysrhythmias.

b. **Management.** To manage a patient with cardiac contusion, you should:

(1) Be alert for possible cardiac arrest.

(2) Help the casualty avoid movement and conditions which could cause a change in heart rate.

(3) Stabilize the patient and evacuate immediately.

c. **Complication--Cardiac Tamponade.**

(1) Cardiac tamponade. Cardiac tamponade, complication of cardiac contusion, is a condition in which blood or other fluid which has leaked out of the heart in the chest injury is caught in the pericardial sac. The fluid accumulates and compresses the heart so that the chambers of the heart can't hold the blood normally returned to it. This situation must be corrected immediately.

(2) Signs/symptoms of cardiac tamponade.

(a) Thready, rapid pulse.

(b) Converging systolic/diastolic blood pressure. (Upper and lower blood pressure readings come closer and closer together as successive readings are taken.)

(c) Distended neck veins.

(d) Muffled heart sounds.

(e) Cool, pale, and clammy skin.

(f) Death may result, due to inadequate cardiac output.

1-9. HEMOTHORAX

Hemothorax is hemorrhaging within the thorax due to the rupture of blood vessels in the chest. The chest is filled up with something other than the lungs. The result is that the lungs cannot expand normally. The casualty is not able to inhale as much air, and there may be less blood to carry this reduced amount of oxygen through the casualty's body. A common cause of hemothorax is a penetrating object to the chest.

a. **Signs/Symptoms of Hemothorax.** Signs and symptoms include the following:

(1) Respiratory difficulty such as dyspnea or gasping respiration.

(2) Decreased, absent, or hyporesonance (dull) respiratory sound.

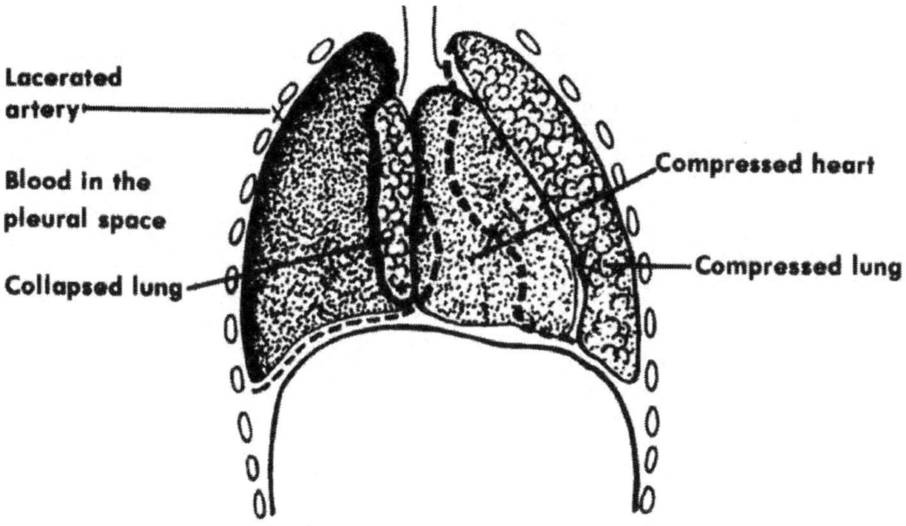

Figure 1-2. Hemothorax.

(3) Early and severe signs of hypovolemia (abnormally diminished volume of blood circulating in the body) and shock to include:

(a) Loss of up to three liters of blood, possibly in a short period of time.

(b) Low blood pressure.

(c) Increased heart rate.

(4) A chest x-ray will show:

(a) Collapse of a lung.

(b) Fluid in the pleural space.

b. **Treatment for Hemothorax.** To treat for hemothorax, you should:

(1) Treat for shock. Follow the general principles of treating for hypovolemic shock (shock caused by diminished blood volume). Start an IV to replace lost body fluid.

(2) Administer oxygen.

c. **Treatment for Hemothorax.** Follow the general principles of treating for hypovolemic shock (shock caused by a decrease in the amount of blood circulating in the body).

(1) Survey the casualty and maintain the airway, if necessary.

(2) Reassure the casualty.

(3) Position the casualty. Place the casualty in the Fowler's position (elevate the casualty's head about 20 inches).

(4) Administer oxygen. Establish an airway (clear the casualty's airway of obstructions and/or secretions and insert an oropharyngeal or endotracheal tube, if necessary). Then administer oxygen by mask or nasal catheter.

(5) Initiate intravenous infusion (IV). Use serum albumin in the IV fluid because serum albumin draws fluid into the tissue. Run the IV flow wide open until the blood pressure returns to normal and stabilizes; then, decrease the flow to one drop per second. Start as many IVs as possible if shock is severe.

(6) Maintain the casualty's normal body temperature. In cool temperatures, place the casualty on a poncho and cover him with the sides of the poncho. Use a wool blanket if you have one. DO NOT allow the casualty to lie in water. In hot or warm temperatures, DO NOT cover the casualty unless he shows signs of chilling. Watch the casualty for signs of sweating and/or chilling. Remove covering if the casualty is sweating. Cover the casualty if he shows signs of chilling.

(7) Check vital signs. Check the casualty's vital signs and other symptoms as often as possible to see if he is responding to treatment. Check for consciousness, blood pressure, pulse rate, respirations, and skin color.

(8) Evacuate the casualty. Record the treatment and evacuate the casualty to the nearest medical facility as soon as possible.

(9) DO NOT drain the pleural space while you are in the field.

1-10. SIMPLE PNEUMOTHORAX

Simple pneumothorax is the presence of air within the pleural space. It results from blunt or penetrating trauma. Ninety percent of such injuries are associated with blunt trauma to the ribs. The fractured rib(s), in turn, cause injury to the pleura.

a. **Signs/Symptoms of Simple Pneumothorax.** Signs and symptoms include the following:

(1) Pain that is sudden and sharp (in spontaneous pneumothorax).

(2) Diminished or absent breath sounds.

(3) Hyperresonance (exaggerated sound) on the affected side as detected by percussion.

(4) Dyspnea (labored breathing) or gasping respiration.

(5) Tracheal deviation toward the affected side.

(6) A dry cough.

b. **Treatment of Simple Pneumothorax.** To treat simple pneumothorax, you should:

(1) Maintain the airway.

(2) Administer oxygen.

(3) If the wound is small, the vital signs are stable, and there is no respiratory distress, transport the casualty in a position that is comfortable for him.

(4) If the wound is large, perform chest decompression. Symptoms of a large wound are:

(a) Marked respiratory distress.

(b) Tachycardia (rapid pulse).

(c) Hypotension (low blood pressure).

1-11. SUBCUTANEOUS EMPHYSEMA

The presence of air or gas in the subcutaneous tissues is called subcutaneous emphysema. This condition can be caused by a blow to the chest which has caused a lung laceration from a fractured rib. If the chest injury is very severe, subcutaneous emphysema can involve the entire chest, neck, and face.

a. **Signs/Symptoms of Subcutaneous Emphysema.** The signs and symptoms include the following:

(1) Soft-tissue crepitus. As you feel over the area of the fracture with your fingertips, you will feel skin that seems like rice krispies.

(2) Occasionally, you will hear crackling sounds when you auscultate the chest.

b. **Treatment of Subcutaneous Emphysema.** To treat subcutaneous emphysema, you should:

(1) Determine the underlying injury--fractured rib, lung laceration, etc.--and treat the injury.

(2) Have the casualty rest.

(3) Monitor respiration.

(4) Administer oxygen. If you use the highest concentration possible, you may reduce the signs and symptoms.

1-12. OPEN PNEUMOTHORAX

Open pneumothorax, also called sucking chest wound, occurs as a result of an external penetrating trauma such as a shotgun wound at close range. The gunshot lacerates (tears) the flesh leaving an open wound. The open wound allows air to enter the chest cavity through the wound each time the casualty inhales and the chest expands in the normal respiratory cycle. In this situation, the air remains outside the lung in the pleural space. When the casualty exhales, air goes back outside through the wound. The lung, due to air in the pleural space, has not been able to fill and function properly.

a. **Signs/Symptoms of Open Pneumothorax.**

(1) Bloody froth in the wound when the casualty breathes out.

(2) A sucking sound at the wound site each time the casualty breathes in.

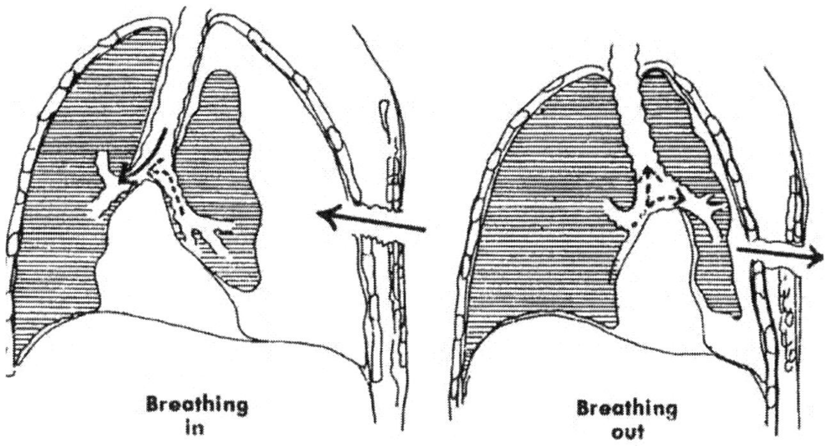

Figure 1-3. Open pneumothorax.

b. **Treatment for Open Pneumothorax.** To treat for open pneumothorax, you should:

(1) Seal the wound immediately with your hand or any available material. The goal is to seal the wound; therefore, use a nonporous material, if possible, such as aluminum foil, or a rolled up 8 x 10 dressing held in place. Be sure the dressing is large enough to cover the wound; otherwise, the dressing might be sucked into the wound.

(2) As soon as possible, apply a petroleum gauze dressing on the wound, and cover the dressing with a bulky dressing taped in place.

(3) Administer oxygen with positive pressure, as needed.

(4) Place the casualty in the semi-Fowler's position or any other position that is comfortable. If he is unconscious, lay him on his injured side.

(5) Observe the casualty for signs and symptoms of shock.

(6) Evacuate the casualty immediately.

(7) Give the casualty an IV with serum albumin.

1-13. TENSION PNEUMOTHORAX

Tension pneumothorax, a complication of hemothorax and pneumothorax, is a type of pneumothorax in which the intra-pleural pressure is greater than the atmospheric pressure. A leak in the lung has occurred, and that leak has failed to seal when the lung collapsed. With every breath the casualty takes, air continuously leaks out of the lung into the chest cavity. The lung collapses more with every breath until finally the lung is a small ball, perhaps two or three inches in diameter. If this condition is not corrected, it will be fatal.

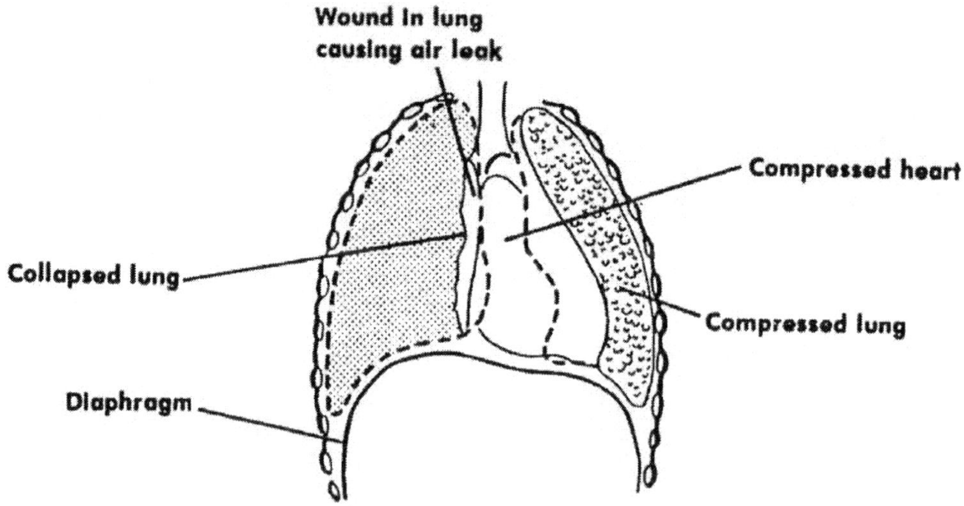

Figure 1-4. Tension pneumothorax.

a. **Characteristics of Tension Pneumothorax.**

(1) The margins or edges of the tear in the pleura are positioned to form a one-way valve. This valve permits air to enter the pleural sac during inspiration (breathing in) but prevents air from escaping during expiration (breathing out) so that each excursion (breath) tends to increase the pressure in the chest. This causes the other lung and the heart to be compressed.

(2) Additionally, the heart and mediastinum are pushed away from the injured side.

(3) Ventilation (air in lungs is exchanged with atmospheric air) and circulation are impaired.

b. **Signs/Symptoms of Tension Pneumothorax.**

(1) Rib fracture or a penetrating wound.

(2) Progressive respiratory distress.

(3) Subcutaneous emphysema. Refer to paragraph 1-11. In this case, there is severe involvement of the entire chest, face, and neck. The area may appear grotesque and/or bloated.

(4) Pain on the affected side.

(5) The affected side will appear more prominent and move less. Air will remain trapped within the pleural cavity on exhalation.

(6) Breath sounds will be distant or absent on the affected side.

(7) Percussion reveals hyperresonance (exaggerated resonance on the affected side).

(8) Progressive distention of the abdomen that is not relieved by gastric aspiration (removal of fluids from the stomach) and endotracheal intubation.

(9) Deep cyanosis (bluish discoloration of the skin caused by insufficient oxygen in the blood).

(10) Shock.

c. **Treatment of Tension Pneumothorax.**

(1) Perform thoracentesis, if required. Thoracentesis is a method of removing air or fluids by suction (aspirating) by surgical puncture of the chest wall into the parietal cavity To perform thoracentesis, follow this procedure:

(a) Gather equipment according to local standing operating procedure (SOP).

(b) Locate the proper site of entry by counting ribs. The site will be high if you are removing air and lower if you are removing fluid. For air, the site of entry is the medclavicular area of the second intercostal space. (The second intercostal space is the space between the second and third ribs). To remove fluid, the site is the intercostal space between the sixth and seventh ribs. To locate the specific ribs, count backward from the twelfth rib (see figure 1-5).

(c) Prep the skin with an antiseptic swab and drape with sterile towels.

(d) Follow local standing operating procedure (SOP) for the complete procedure.

(e) Aspirate air or fluid from the chest cavity. Continue aspiration until there is no more air or fluid to remove <u>or</u> until over 500 ml of blood or 1000 ml of air have been removed. A tube thoracostomy (a surgical creation of an opening into the chest wall) is usually performed when the casualty is evacuated to a treatment facility.

(2) Perform chest decompression.

(a) For closed injuries, insert a large bore needle into the second incostal (ICS) mid-clavicular line (MCL). The plunger rises on its own when under pressure.

(b) For an open injury, cover the injury with a dressing and periodically remove the dressing to let air escape.

(3) Perform a tube thoracostomy using the second incostal mid-clavicular line. This procedure is a must if the casualty is to be air-transported.

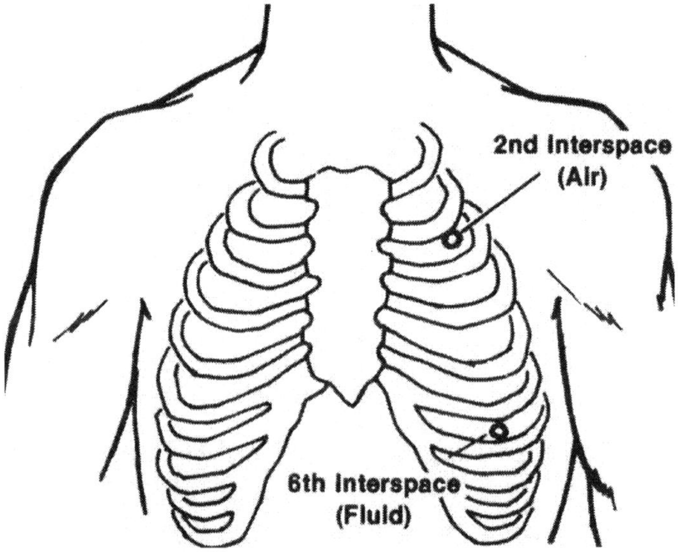

Figure 1-5. Needle insertion site for tension pneumothorax.

(4) Give the highest concentration of oxygen possible. Use positive pressure as needed. The positive pressure may increase tension; however, if decompression has been accomplished (air removed from the chest cavity), the lungs may expand.

(5) Place the casualty in the Fowler's position, as tolerated.

(6) Start an IV using normal saline or Ringer's solution.

(7) Monitor the casualty's cardiac rhythm.

Section III. CHEST DECOMPRESSION

1-14. GENERAL INFORMATION

Chest decompression is the removal of air or blood from the chest cavity through a seal or valve device. Once the chest cavity is emptied of air or blood, the lung can expand and pressure in the chest cavity once again becomes negative.

a. **Indications of Need for Chest Decompression.**Any casualty with one of the following chest injuries will probably need chest decompression:

(1) Tension pneumothorax (collapsed lung).

(2) Hemothorax (accumulation of blood in the pleural cavity).

(3) Simple pneumothorax (accumulation of air in the thorax), if the wound is large.

(4) Flail chest with pneumothorax.

b. **Complications Associated with Chest Decompression.** Complications which may occur include the following:

(1) Bleeding from the intercostal artery.

(2) Lung puncture.

(3) Hitting a pulmonary vessel.

1-15. NEEDLE CHEST DECOMPRESSION

a. **Symptoms**. Needle chest decompression is indicated if one of the following conditions exists: the casualty has tension pneumothorax; air must be released from the casualty's chest and adequate instruments are not available; the casualty has massive pneumothorax with mediastinal shift or without mediastinal shift.

b. **Procedures for Needle Chest Decompression.** To perform a needle chest decompression, complete the following steps taking care NOT to injure the casualty further.

(1) Gather equipment. You will need the following items:

(a) Stethoscope.

(b) Large bore needle (12 to 14 gauge).

(c) 30 to 50 ml syringe.

(d) Iodine swab.

(e) DD Form 1380 (Field Medical Card).

(f) Pencil.

(2) Verify the presence of pneumothorax. Do this by checking for indications of the condition.

CAUTION: Correct assessment is essential. If a needle is inserted into a normal chest, the casualty will almost certainly develop pneumothorax.

(a) Ask the casualty if there is a sharp pain on the affected side. Ask for any information related to the condition; for example, pain, trauma, or difficulty in breathing.

(b) Look for signs and symptoms of shock--decreased temperature; weak, thready pulse; rapid, shallow respirations; etc.

(c) Check for lack of chest excursion by observing the rising and falling of the chest during the casualty's respirations. Also, compare chest excursion on both sides of the chest to see if the chest rises and falls equally on both sides.

(d) Look for mediastinal (the mass of organs and tissues separating the two lungs) shift. Two signs of mediastinal shift are a tracheal deviation and/or distention of the jugular vein.

(e) Look for unilateral distention (change affecting one side) in this manner:

1 Place one hand on the affected area.

2 Place the other hand on the unaffected side.

3 Observe the height of each hand.

4 Determine if the height of the hand on the affected side is greater during expiration than the height of the hand on the unaffected side.

(f) Look and listen for the casualty gasping for air (dyspnea).Dyspnea may be present, but is not always an indication of pneumothorax.

(g) Look at and feel the casualty's chest for signs of subcutaneous emphysema.

(h) Tap the chest for tympany (a sound heard when percussing the chest). Percuss the chest in this manner:

1 Position the middle finger of one hand on the superior portion of the unaffected side.

2 Sharply tap the positioned finger with the middle finger of the other hand.

3 Repeat the previous two steps and listen for tympany on the affected side.

4 Repeat tapping the chest for tympany in successively lower positions on the chest until the entire chest has been percussed.

(i) Listen for diminished breath sounds.

1 Place the stethoscope on the unaffected side to establish normal breath sounds.

2 Listen to the affected side to determine if the breath sounds are fainter. The pneumothorax may be bilateral (affecting both sides of the chest).

(3) Locate the insertion site.

(a) Locate the sternomanubrial joint (Angle of Louis).

(b) Start at the sternomanubrial joint and follow the adjacent intercostal space to the mid-clavicular line.

(4) Clean the insertion site.

(a) Remove the swab from the wrapper.

(b) Clean from the insertion site outward in a circular motion for 3 to 4 inches.

(5) Insert the needle with the attached syringe.

(a) Place the needle tip, bevel up, on the insertion site, centered on the third rib.

(b) Lower the proximal end of the needle to permit the tip to enter the skin over the third rib.

(c) Insert the needle into the skin over the third rib until you have penetrated the pleura. When the pleura is penetrated, you will feel a "POP" followed by expulsion of air through the needle.

(6) Aspirate air. Aspirate as much air as necessary to relieve the patient's acute symptoms.

CAUTION: Avoid puncturing blood vessels and nerves!

(7) Withdraw the needle.

(a) Look for signs of respiratory relief as evidenced by the absence of the symptoms of pneumothorax.

(b) Withdraw the needle along the angle of insertion.

(8) Record. If you are in a field setting, record the treatment on the Field Medical Card.

1-16. CATHETER-OVER-NEEDLE CHEST DECOMPRESSION

Perform a catheter-over-needle chest decompression. To do this procedure correctly, you must perform the following steps in sequence being careful not to cause further injury to the casualty.

a. Gather your equipment. You will need the following items:

(1) Stethoscope.

(2) Catheter-over-needle device (12 to 14 gauge).

(3) Iodine swab.

(4) Adhesive tape, 6 inches of 1/2 inch wide tape.

(5) DD Form 1380 (Field Medical Card.)

(6) Pencil.

b. Verify the presence of pneumothorax by checking for indications of this chest injury. Follow the same verification procedures as for needle chest decompression listed in paragraphs 1-15a(2)(a) through 1-15a(3)(a)(i).

c. Locate the insertion site. Follow procedure explained in 1-15a(3)(a) and (b).

d. Clean the insertion site as in 15a(4)(a) and (b).

e. Insert the needle.

(1) Place the needle tip, bevel up, on the insertion site, centered on the third rib.

(2) Lower the proximal end of the needle to permit the tip to enter the skin over the third rib.

(3) Insert the needle into the skin over the third rib, until the pleura has been penetrated, as evidenced by feeling a "POP", followed by expulsion of air through the needle.

(4) Hold the exposed end of the needle so it will NOT move.

f. Push the catheter into the pleural space until you feel resistance when the catheter meets the apex of the lungs.

g. While you keep the catheter from moving, withdraw the needle along the angle of insertion.

h. Secure the catheter to the chest.

i. If you are in a field situation, record the treatment on the Field Medical Card.

Continue with Exercises

EXERCISES, LESSON 1

INSTRUCTIONS. Answer the following exercises by writing the answer in the space provided.

After you have completed all of these exercises, turn to "Solutions to Exercises" at the end of the lesson and check your answers. For each exercise answered incorrectly, reread the material referenced with the solution.

1. List three common causes (listed in this lesson) of penetrating/nonpenetrating chest injuries.

   a. ____.

   b. ____.

   c. ____.

2. List four common signs/symptoms of chest injuries.

   a. ____.

   b. ____.

   c. ____.

   d. ____.

3. When you examine a casualty to detect a chest injury, you should:

   a. Question the casualty if he is.____________________

   b. Observe the casualty's bare chest and upper abdomen for __________ and depth.

   c. Check for ______________________ on both sides of the chest.

   d. Examine the ______________________(including the back) beneath any overlying clothing.

   e. Listen to the casualty's chest near the _______________and compare

   both sides of the chest for ___________, _____________, and equality

4. Rib and sternum damage, flail chest, and cardiac contusion are examples of

_________________________ chest injuries.

5. A penetrating chest injury may be a hole in the thoracic cavity that allows

___________________________________.

6. Follow these general principles of treatment for chest trauma:

   a. Keep the pleural space _________________by suctioning, if necessary.

   b. Give oxygen to maintain proper level of oxygen in the body and to

   _________________________________.

   c. Estimate the amount of hemorrhage the casualty has, and

   _____________________________________.

   d. Suction to keep the bronchial tree clear of retained blood,

   _______________________________, and bronchial secretions.

7. ______________________ is a chest injury in which the pressure in the pleural cavity is greater than the atmospheric pressure.

8. A casualty with a chest injury is experiencing paradoxical respirations (the chest expands when he exhales and the chest contracts when he inhales). The name of the chest injury is probably _________________________________.

9. List two indications for needle chest decompression.

a. ____.

b. ____.

10. The needle used for a needle chest decompression is a _____________ needle.

11. Insertion of a needle into the pleural space of a casualty who does not have pneumothorax will result in the person having ________________________.

12. When tapping the chest for tympany, you should use the middle finger of one hand and ______________________________ of the other hand.

13. When performing a needle chest decompression, insert the needle

____

Check Your Answers on Next Page

SOLUTIONS TO EXERCISES, LESSON 1

1. You are correct if you listed any three of the following:

   Automobile accidents.
   Falls.
   Gunshot wounds.
   Stab wounds.
   Crushing injuries. (para 1-1)

2. You are correct if you listed any four of the following:

   Normal breathing pattern change.
   Pain at injury site.
   Dyspnea (shortness of breath).
   Chest doesn't expand.
   Rapid/weak pulse.
   Low blood pressure.
   Dry or bloody cough.
   Sucking sound on respiration.
   Cyanosis.
   Hemoptysis. (paras 1-2a through 1-2j)

3. a. conscious

   b. Respiratory rate.

   c. Equal movement.

   d. Entire chest wall.

   e. Armpits, volume, loudness. (paras 1-3a through 1-3e)

4. Blunt. (paras 1-6a, 1-7, 1-8)

5. Air enter the thorax thus filling that cavity with air. (para 1-4a)

6. a. Empty.

   b. Remove carbon dioxide.

   c. Replace the blood as necessary.

   d. Foreign material. (paras 1-5a through 5e)

7. Tension pneumothorax. (para 1-13)

8. Flail chest. (para 1-7a)

9. You are correct if you listed any two of the following:

   . Casualty has tension pneumothorax.
   . Casualty needs emergency release of air from the pleural cavity and adequate instruments are not available.
   . Casualty has massive pneumothorax with or without mediastinal shift.
   (para 1-15a)

10. 12 to 14 gauge large bore. (paras 1-15b(1)(b)

11. Pneumothorax. (para 1-15b(2) CAUTION)

12. The middle finger. (paras 1-15b(2)(h) 1, 2.)

13. Into the skin over the third rib. (para 1-15b(5)(c)

End of Lesson 1

LESSON ASSIGNMENT

LESSON 2 Airway Management.

LESSON ASSIGNMENT Paragraphs 2-1 through 2-13.

LESSON OBJECTIVES After completing this lesson, you should be able to:

2-1. State the purpose of using an esophageal obturator airway (EOA) or an esophageal gastric tube airway (EGTA).

2-2. Identify the advantages/ disadvantages of using an EOA or an EGTA.

2-3. Identify the indications/ contraindications of using an EOA or an EGTA.

2-4. Place the steps of intubating with an EOA or an EGTA in the correct order of performance.

2-5. Place the steps of extubating an EOA or an EGTA in the correct order of performance.

2-6. Identify the advantages/disadvantages of using an endotracheal tube (ET).

2-7. Identify the indications/contraindications of using an ET.

2-8. Place the steps for intubating with an ET in the correct order of performance.

2-9. Place the steps for extubating an ET in the correct order of performance.

SUGGESTION After completing the assignment, complete the exercises of this lesson. These exercises will help you to achieve the lesson objectives.

Section I. ESOPHAGEAL OBTURATOR AIRWAY

2-1. INTRODUCTION

Intubation, a valuable technique, is used frequently in the administration of anesthesia, cardiopulmonary resuscitation, and respiratory therapy. The procedure improves safety by establishing and maintaining the casualty's airway, allowing the surgeon greater freedom of access to the operative field, and improving aseptic technique for head and neck surgery. However, the procedure requires both a knowledgeable and skillful medical specialist. The esophageal obturator airway (EOA) is a long tube open at the top, sealed at the bottom, with numerous side holes near its upper end. The esophageal gastric tube airway (EGTA) is a variation of the EOA. It has no holes on the tube, but the tip of the obturator is open rather than closed. The technique for passing (inserting) the EOA and the EGTA are the same. Neither the EOA nor the EGTA provides the perfect answer to controlling the airway and neither should be considered as replacements for endotracheal intubation (ET). Their most appropriate use is as an interim form of airway control in patients who are difficult to intubate endotracheally.

2-2. PURPOSE OF THE EOA AND EGTA

The esophageal obturator airway and the esophageal gastric tube airway have several important purposes. Each device, when inserted, holds the tongue away from the pharynx allowing ventilated air to move through the trachea into the lungs. Additionally, the EOA and the EGTA, when inserted, seal off the stomach from the airway thus preventing gastric acid from coming back into the pharynx. The EGTA can be used for gastric lavage (washing out the stomach) and gavage (forced feeding by flexible tube and pump).

2-3. ADVANTAGES/DISADVANTAGES OF THE EOA AND EGTA

a. **Advantages of EOA and EGTA.** There are two main advantages in using these devices. First, both the EOA and the EGTA are easy to place. Second, only minimal training is required to learn to place the devices properly.

b. **Disadvantages of EOA and EGTA.** These are the disadvantages. Theses devices DO NOT allow a direct pathway into the larynx for suctioning. The mask face seal must be good for ventilation. It is possible to cause pharyngeal trauma to the patient during insertion of the device. It is possible to accidentally enter the trachea and totally obstruct the airway. Finally, if the cuff of the EOA is not properly inflated, gastric distention and impaired ventilation can be caused. Neither of these devices should be used on anyone less than five feet tall; the tubes are too long for people of such height.

2-4. INDICATIONS/CONTRAINDICATIONS OF THE EOA AND EGTA

a. **Indications for Use of the EOA and EGTA.** Either of these devices can be used if one of the following conditions exist: the casualty is in a deep coma; the casualty has shallow respirations; the casualty has progressive cyanosis; the casualty has cardiopulmonary arrest.

NOTE: The EGTA may be used for gastric lavage (washing out of the stomach) or gavage (forced feeding by flexible tube and pump) which might be required for a patient who has taken an overdose of drugs.

b. **Contraindications for Use of EOA and EGTA.** These devices should not be used if these conditions exist. Do not use if the casualty is conscious and/or is breathing effectively on his own. The gag reflex may operate causing the casualty to retch or choke. Do not use either device on infants, children, or adults under five feet tall. Devices small enough to fit these individuals have not been developed. Do not use EOAs or EGTAs if the casualty has facial damage, esophageal disease, or if the casualty has ingested a caustic substance.

2-5. INTUBATING WITH AN EOA AND EGTA

a. **Equipment.** The following equipment will be needed to perform an EOA or ETGA intubation:

(1) Esophageal obturator airway (EOA or EGTA)

(2) 50 cc syringe.

(3) Lubricating jelly (K-Y or Lidocaine Jelly).

(4) EGTA (gastric tube).

(5) EOA (suction device).

b. **Procedural Steps for Intubating.** Complete the following steps:

(1) Gather the equipment:

(a) EOA or EGTA syringe.

(b) K-Y lubricant.

(c) Bag-valve-mask (BVM) or oxygen with demand valve. Check the BVM each time prior to use, particularly the cuff. Also, check the corneal reflex and the gag reflex. Check the casualty for the presence of a corneal reflex by touching the casualty's cornea with your fingers. If the eyelid does not try to close, continue with the procedure. If the eyelid tries to close (blink), the gag reflex is still present and you cannot proceed with insertion of the device. Periodically recheck for the reflex, and when the eyelid does not try to close, continue with the procedure.

(2) Lubricate the EOA or EGTA.

(3) Oxygenate the casualty with two full, slow breaths.

(4) Grasp the casualty's tongue and jaw, lifting both upward and forward without hyperextending the neck.

(5) Grasp the tube below the mask using the fingers of your other hand.

(6) Insert the EOA or EGTA (without pushing hard) following the curve of the pharynx until the mask settles on the casualty's face.

(7) Seal the mask and check its placement by blowing into the tube and watching for the rise of the casualty's. (If the chest does not expand or rise, remove the tube quickly and reoxygenate.)

NOTE: You must wait 3 minutes before doing these procedures again.

(8) Inflate the balloon of the EOA or EGTA with no more than 35 ml of air.

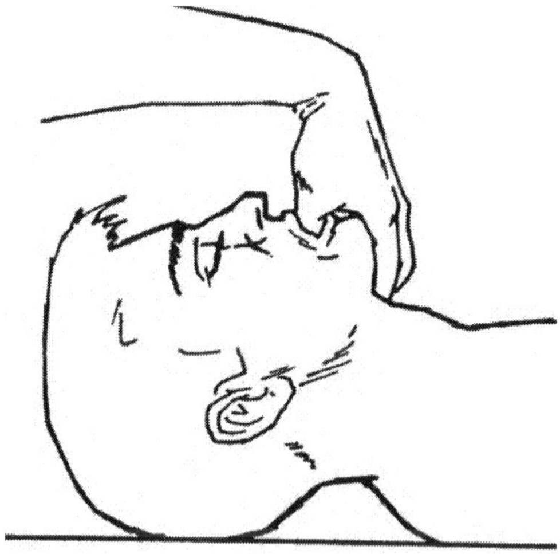

Figure 2-1. Grasp the casualty's tongue and jaw.

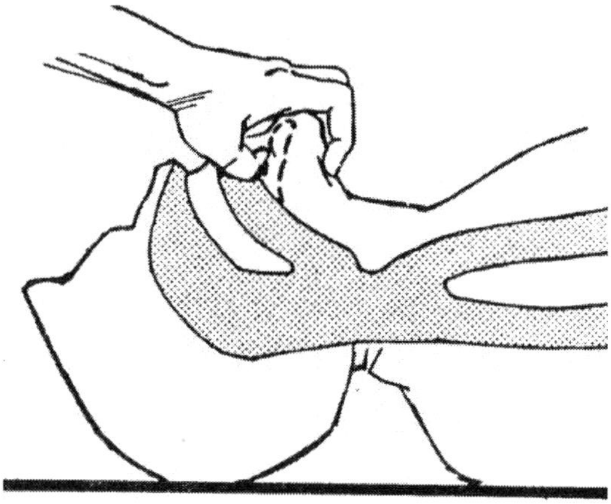

Figure 2-2. Lift the tongue and jaw upward.

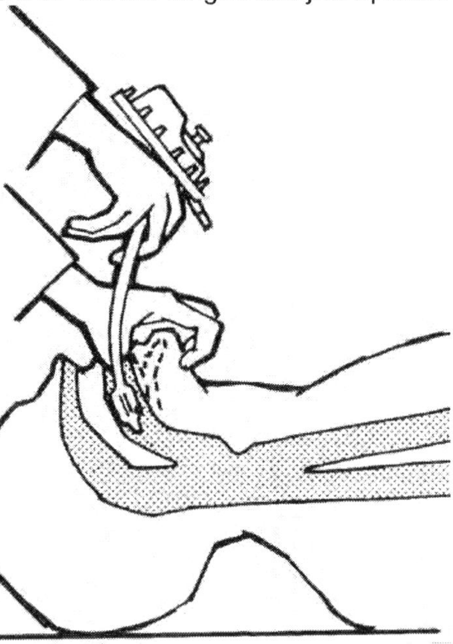

Figure 2-3. Insert the EOA or EGTA tip into the mouth.

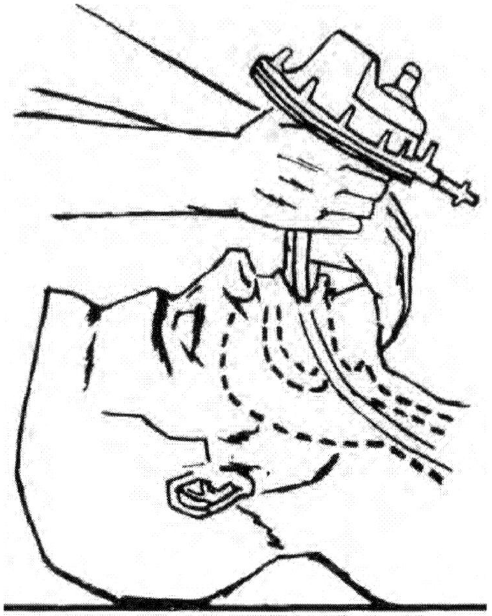

Figure 2-4. Continue inserting the EOA or EGTA following the curve of the pharynx.

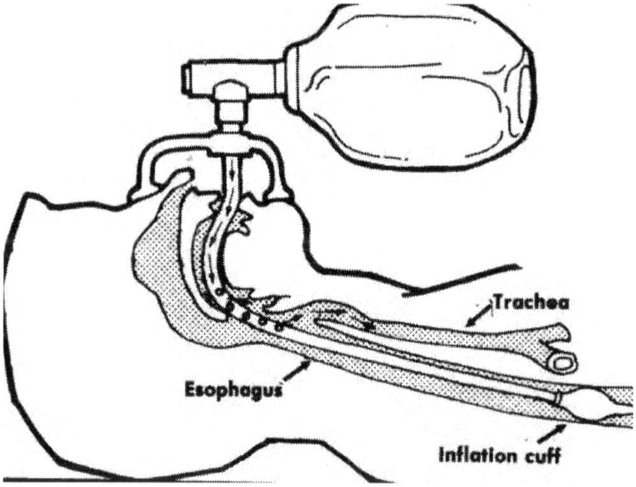

Figure 2-5. Inflate the balloon of the EOA or EGTA.

(9) Remove the syringe to allow self-sealing or clamp the cuff tube, if necessary.

(10) Auscultate to check placement of the EOA or EGTA by listening with a stethoscope to the two lower lung fields and the paraumbilical area. You should not hear a sound like rushing water.

(11) Ventilate once every 5 seconds using a bag-valve-mask (BMV) or a demand valve and oxygen.

NOTE: At any point during the procedure, the casualty should NOT be without oxygen for more than 30 seconds

2-6. EXTBATING WITH AN EOA AND EGTA

CAUTION: The EOA or EGTA is not normally removed until the casualty is in the hospital unless the casualty begins to breathe on his own.

Follow these steps to extubate (remove) an EOA or an EGTA:

a. Oxygenate the casualty with two slow breaths. You can do this by blowing two slow breaths into the tube, or you can attach an ambu bag and squeeze it two times. What you are doing is giving the casualty a little too much oxygen to compensate for the time when he will not be getting quite enough oxygen--the time you are removing the EOA or the EGTA.

b. Pop off the face mask.

c. Turn the patient to one side.

d. Deflate the balloon cuff with the syringe.

e. Remove the tube following the curve of the pharynx.

f. Clear the airway of vomitus immediately.

Section II. ENDOTRACHEAL TUBE

2-7. INTRODUCTION

An endotracheal tube (ET) is a tube inserted into the trachea for administration of anesthesia, maintenance of an airway, aspirations of secretions, ventilation of the lungs, or prevention of the entrance of foreign material into the tracheobronchial tree. The two types of ETs dealt with in this lesson are the orotracheal tube and the nasotracheal tube. The orotracheal tube is inserted through the mouth into the trachea. The nasotracheal tube is inserted through the nose into the trachea. In this lesson, both the orotracheal tube and the nasotracheal tube are used to establish an airway.

2-8. ADVANTAGES/DISADVANTAGES OF ET

a. **Advantages of ET.** The chief advantage is that the endotracheal tube provides an unobstructed airway if the tube is properly placed. Air is channeled through the larynx and trachea to the lungs where it is needed. In normal breathing, some air breathed remains in the larynx and trachea where the air is unused. The space holding the unused air is called anatomic dead space, and the endotracheal tube reduces that space by about 50 percent. Once inserted, the ET prevents the casualty from breathing in secretions such as blood, stomach contents and bowel contents. The ET also makes positive pressure breathing (assisted or controlled) easier without gastric inflation.

b. **Disadvantages of ET.** With the ET in place, air goes directly through the mouth without being warmed, humidified, or filtered--all of which normally take place in the nasal passages. It is possible to cause further injury to the casualty by accidentally inserting the tube into the wrong area. A tube inserted into the esophagus, for example, can cause the airway to be completely obstructed. Also, the presence of the tube may be such an irritant to the casualty's body that he may have breathing problems. The tube may cause bronchial spasms or increase the production of mucous, both make it more difficult for air to reach the casualty's lungs.

2-9. INDICATIONS/CONTRAINDICATIONS FOR USE OF ET

a. **Indications.** Indications for using the endotracheal tube are the same as for using the esophageal obturator airway--casualty in deep coma, casualty with shallow respirations, casualty has progressive cyanosis, or casualty has cardiopulmonary arrest. Additionally, use the ET when preparing a person before surgery for anesthesia. The ET is used in all types of surgery where the casualty's position makes it impossible to use a mask; for example, the prone (lying face downward), lateral (lying on side with top knee bent for balance), or sitting positions. The ET is used if a tight mask fit is not possible due to "atypical" (abnormal) facial contours caused by disease, obesity, etc.

b. **Contraindications.** Don't use the endotracheal tube if there is upper airway obstruction due to foreign bodies. Use the endotracheal tube with caution if there is swelling in the larynx or if the patient has mandibular (horseshoe-shaped bone forming the lower jaw) or cervical (neck) fractures. Attempts at intubation may make these injuries worse.

2-10. INTUBATING WITH AN ET

a. **Equipment.** Endotracheal tubes are nontoxic, nonallergenic, and flexible. These tubes are able to maintain a curved shape and do not conduct electricity. There are two types of tubes: rubber tubes and plastic tubes. Rubber tubes include the Murphy, a blunt level type of endotracheal tube with an inflatable cuff. The Cole, a pediatric tube, is also made of rubber. Plastic tubes, can be either opaque or transparent; the Protex is an example of such a tube. The Protex tube is made of transparent vinyl plastic; the tube tends to bend although it is somewhat rigid.

(1) Tube size.

(a) Measure the external diameter of the tube in millimeters.

(b) The internal diameter is measured in millimeters. The internal diameter size is basically standard but may vary to about 0.5mm.

(c) To determine the length of the oral tube, measure the distance from the corner of the casualty's mouth to midsternum (mid breast bone).

(d) The casualty's nare size will determine the nasal tube's diameter. To determine the length of the nasal tube, measure the distance from the earlobe to the corner of the mouth and add the distance from the corner of the mouth to the midsternum. The radius of the curvature is greater for oral tubes. The bevel for the nasal tube has a sharper angle than for the oral tubes. There is also a difference in the inflatable cuffs.

(2) Inflatable cuffs. These are used to attain an airtight seal to prevent aspiration. The cuffs should be inflated so the balloon indents with thumb pressure. Such indentation usually occurs when the balloon has been inflated with five to ten milliliters of air.

(3) Stylet. The stylet allows the proper tube curvature to be maintained.

(4) Magill forceps. These are used to guide the nasal endotracheal tube into the larynx from the pharynx.

(5) Laryngoscope. This device is used to see the larynx. A laryngoscope has two different types of blades: the Miller blade which is straight and the MacIntosh blade which is curved. The component parts are:

(a) Handle ("L" type or right angle is the most commonly used handle). Handles come in small, medium, and large sizes.

(b) Flashlight and penlight batteries.

(c) A blade that snaps onto the handle.

b. **Complications.**

(1) In the process of inserting the tube, teeth may be broken or chipped; nasal, oral, and pharyngeal soft tissue may be damaged; or the vocal cord may be damaged.

(2) The tube may be accidentally pushed into the esophagus causing a total airway obstruction and finally death, if the situation is not corrected.

(3) If the tube is pushed into the bronchus (either of the two main branches of the trachea), the casualty may suffer pneumothorax, bronchospasm, laryngospasm, hypoxemia, cardiac arrhythmias, or irritation of the carina with subsequent coughing.

(4) Endotracheal tube obstruction. Foreign bodies, mucous, etc. may block the tube.

(5) The trachea or vocal cords may become ulcerated because of increased pressure by the ET cuff.

(6) After the endotracheal tube is removed, the casualty may experience laryngospasm (spasmodic closure of the larynx), infection, and hoarseness (sore throat).

2-11. PROCEDURAL STEPS FOR INTUBATING--OROTRACHEAL TUBE

Complete the following steps to intubate correctly:

a. Gather the equipment and check it.

(1) Tube. Select the type (vinyl, rubber, or plastic) and the size of the tube. Use anatomy considerations and measurements in your selection. (The inflatable cuff comes with the tube.)

(2) Stylet.

(3) Magill forceps. These forceps can be used to advance the tube between the vocal cords.

(4) Laryngoscope. Check this instrument for batteries and check the light. Select the blade you are going to use and assemble the blade. (The curved blade provides more working space, but the straight blade allows you to see better.)

(5) Suction apparatus with a tonsillar tip.

(6) J-tube (oropharyngeal) airway. A J-tube is a white plastic or black rubber tube that is used to keep the tongue out of the way.

(7) Anesthetic spray, if available.

b. Place the equipment next to the casualty's head, where the equipment is needed.

c. Position the casualty so that you have the best possible view of the larynx. The casualty should be in a "sniffing" position with a towel under his neck.

d. Turn on the suction apparatus.

NOTE: OPTIONAL PROCEDURE--place a stylet into the tube prior to oxygenation and insertion of the laryngoscope.

e. Check the casualty's corneal reflex and his gag reflex, then oxygenate the casualty with two slow breaths. Check the casualty for the presence of a corneal reflex by touching the casualty's cornea with your fingers. If the eyelid does not try to close, continue with the procedure. If the eyelid tries to close (blink), the gag reflex is still present, and you cannot proceed with insertion of the device. Periodically recheck for the reflex, and when the eyelid does not try to close, continue with the procedure.

f. Insert the laryngoscope and place the tube.

(1) Grasp the laryngoscope with your left hand.

(2) Insert the laryngoscope into the right side of the casualty's mouth.

(3) Bring the blade to the center or midline of the mouth, moving the tongue to the left side.

(4) Advance the blade a short distance.

(5) Visualize the epiglottis.

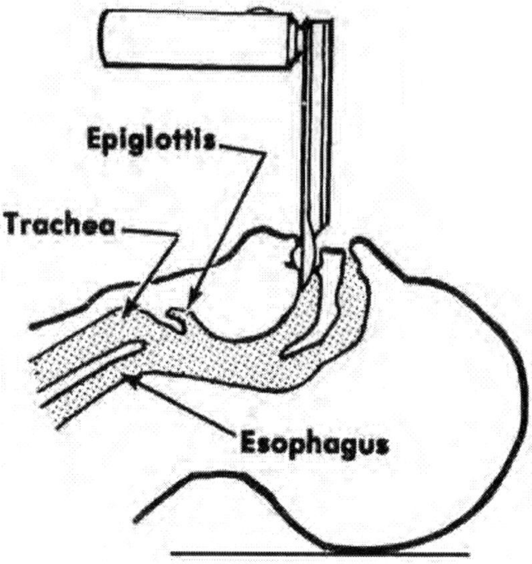

Figure 2-6. Placement of the laryngoscope.

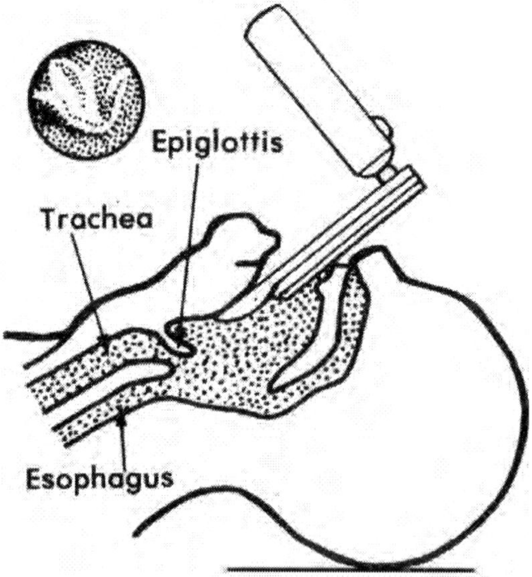

Figure 2-7. Visualization of the epiglottis.

(6) Advance the tip of the blade and lift it to visualize the vocal cords. If you are using a straight blade, place the tip of the blade under the epiglottis. If you are using a curved blade, put the tip of the blade on the vallecula (depression between the epiglottis and the root of the tongue, either side of the median glossoepiglottic fold).

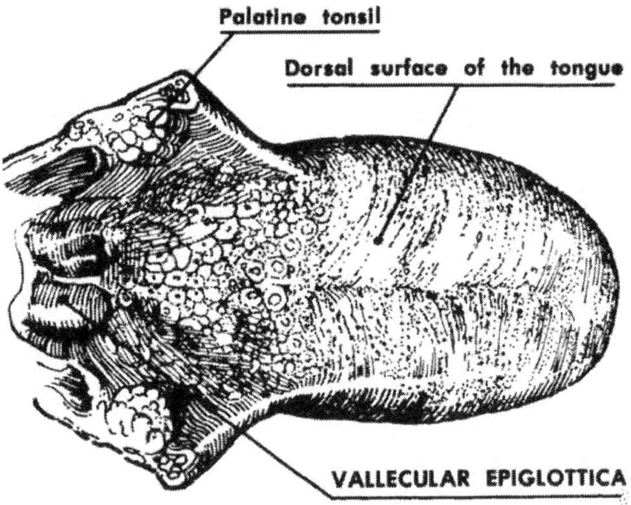

Figure 2-8. Vallecula epiglottica.

(7) Grasp the tube with the right hand.

(8) Advance the tip of the endotracheal tube carefully between the vocal cords until the upper cuff is below the level of the vocal cords.

(9) Insert the oropharyngeal airway (J-tube) to act as a bite block.

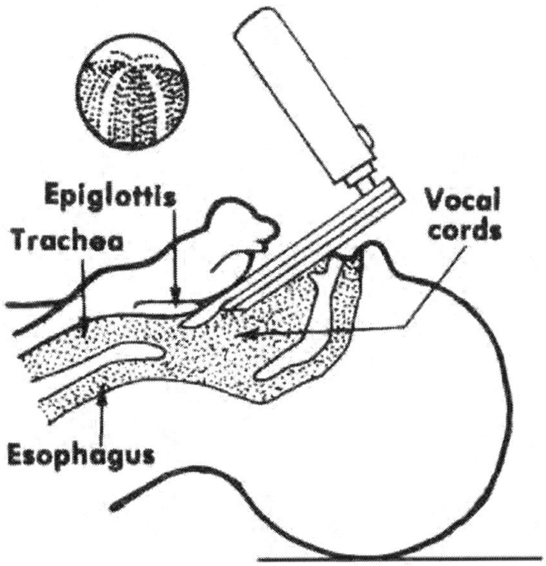

Figure 2-9. Visualization of the vocal cords.

g. Check the placement of the endotracheal tube. To check the placement:

(1) Breathe through the tube while someone auscultates the two lower lung fields and the paraumbilical (area alongside the navel) regions to check tube placement.

(2) If sound is heard over one lung field (usually the right) more than the other, you must back up the tube a little and listen again?

<u>NOTE</u>: If a rushing sound is heard over the abdomen with diffuse sound over the lower lung fields, you have missed the larynx and gone down into the pharynx. You should remove the tube, reoxygenate the casualty, wait three minutes, and try again.

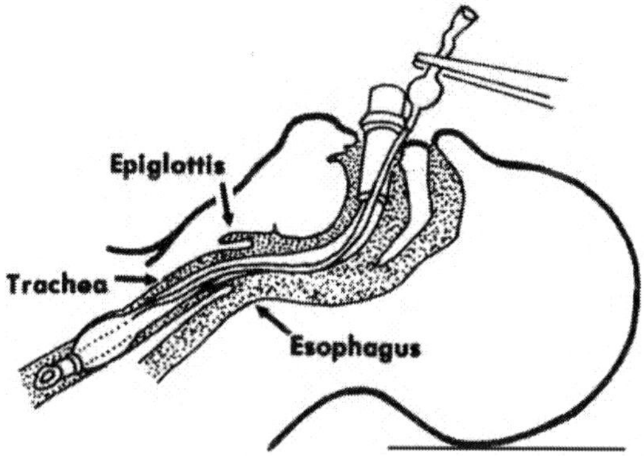

Figure 2-10. Properly placed endotracheal tube.

h. Inflate the cuff with 5 to 10 ml of air.

i. Reoxygenate the patient with two slow breaths.

j. Clamp the tube (optional) and remove the syringe.

k. Connect the resuscitative equipment (BVM or 0_2 with demand valve).

l. Ventilate once every 5 seconds.

m. Secure the tube.

n. Monitor the casualty periodically with auscultation to be sure the endotracheal tube is placed correctly.

CAUTION: Be sure the casualty is NOT without oxygen for longer than 30 seconds at a time.

2-12. PROCEDURAL STEPS FOR INTUBATING--NASOTRACHEAL TUBE

a. Intubate with a nasotracheal tube in the same way as you would with an orotracheal tube. There are some differences, and these differences are listed here.

b. Use the most patent nare. That is, insert the tube in the nostril which is the most open.

c. Advance the tube while you listen to breath sounds.

d. Use the Magill forceps to advance the tube into the larynx. Begin using the forceps when the tube appears in the oropharynx.

e. Be sure the bevel of the tube is adjacent to the nasal septum when the tube is being advanced.

f. Tape the tube across the casualty's nose and cheek on the side that is used.

2-13. EXTUBATING AN ET

The procedure is the same for the nasotracheal tube and the orotracheal tube. Follow these steps:

a. Suction the bronchial tree as required:

(1) Initiate cardiac monitoring.

(2) Preoxygenate for at least 3 minutes.

(3) Advance the catheter as far as possible with the suction off.

(4) Apply intermittent suction while slowly withdrawing the catheter in a rotating fashion.

(5) DO NOT apply suction for more than 5 seconds.

b. Reoxygenate the patient with two slow breaths.

c. Deflate the cuff using the syringe.

d. Remove the tube at the end of inspiration (inhaling).

e. Clear and maintain an open (patent) airway.

Continue with Exercises

EXERCISES, LESSON 2

INSTRUCTIONS. Answer the following exercises by writing the answer in the space provided.

After you have completed all of these exercises, turn to "Solutions to Exercises" at the end of the lesson and check your answers. For each exercise answered incorrectly, reread the material referenced with the solution.

1. List three purposes of the esophageal obturator airway (EOA) and the esophageal gastric tube airway (EGTA).

   a. ______________________________.

   b. ______________________________.

   c. ______________________________.

2. List the two main advantages of using the EOA or the EGTA.

   a. ______________________________.

   b. ______________________________.

3. List three conditions in which you would not use an EOA or EGTA.

   a. ______________________________.

   b. ______________________________.

   c. ______________________________.

4. Just before grasping the casualty's tongue and jaw (in the process of intubating with an EOA or EGTA, you should oxygenate the casualty with ____________ full breaths.

5. During the time you are intubating with an EOA or EGTA, be sure the casualty is not without oxygen more than ______________________________.

6. One possible complication of using an endotracheal tube is that the casualty may develop ______________________________ of the trachea or vocal cords.

7. When you are inserting the EOA or EGTA, insert the tube following the curve of the pharynx until ______________________________.

8. To seal the mask of an EOA or EGTA and check that the tube is properly placed, blow into the tube and watch for ______________________________.

9. The chief advantage of the endotracheal tube, if properly placed, is that it provides ______________________________.

10. If an endotracheal tube is in the casualty, air goes directly through the mouth and is not warmed, ____________________, or __________________ functions normally performed by the nasal passages.

11. When you are using an endotracheal tube, determine the length of the tube by measuring the distance from the casualty's ______________________ and adding the distance from ______________________________.

12. It is possible to cause damage when inserting an endotracheal tube; for example, teeth may be __________________ or ______________________.

13. You are intubating with an orotracheal ET and hear a rushing sound over the abdomen along with sounds over the lower lung fields. You have missed the ____________________ and gone into the ______________________.

14. When intubating with an orotracheal ET, be sure the casualty does not go without oxygen for more than ____________________________ at a time.

15. When intubating with a nasotracheal ET, be sure the ___________________of the tube is adjacent to the nasal septum when the tube is being advanced.

Check Your Answers on Next Page

SOLUTIONS TO EXERCISES, LESSON 2

1. You are correct if you listed any three of the following:

   Each device holds the tongue away from the pharynx, allowing ventilated air to move into the trachea.
   Each device seals off the stomach from the airway, preventing gastric acid from coming back into the pharynx.
   Each device can be used for gastric lavage (irrigation of the stomach).
   Each device can be used for gavage (feeding through a tube passed into the stomach). (para 2-2)

2. The devices are easy to place.
   Only a minimal amount of training is needed to use the devices. (para 2-3a)

3. You are correct if you listed any three of the following:

   The casualty is conscious and breathing effectively on his own.
   The casualty is an infant.
   The casualty is an adult under 5 feet tall.
   The casualty has facial damage.
   The casualty has esophageal disease.
   The casualty has ingested a caustic substance. (para 2-4b)

4. two. (para 2-5b(3))

5. 30 seconds. (para 2-5b(11))

6. Ulceration. (para 2-10b)

7. The mask settles on the casualty's face. (para 2-5b(6))

8. The rise of the casualty's chest. (para 2-5b(7))

9. An unobstructed airway. (para 2-8a)

10. Humidified, or filtered. (para 2-8b)

11. Earlobe to the corner of the mouth.
    Corner of the casualty's mouth to the midsternum. (para 2-10a(1)(d))

12. Chipped or broken. (para 2-1Ob(1))

13. Larynx.
    Pharynx. (para 2-11g(2) NOTE)

14. 30 seconds. (para 2-11n CAUTION)

15. Bevel. (para 2-12e)

End of Lesson 2

LESSON ASSIGNMENT

LESSON 3 Circothyroidotomy

LESSON ASSIGNMENT Paragraphs 3-1 through 3-9.

LESSON OBJECTIVES After completing this lesson, you should be able to:

3-1. Define cricothyroidotomy.

3-2. Identify conditions requiring a cricothyroidotomy, types of cricothyroidotomy, and complications of cricothyroidotomy.

3-3. Identify signs/symptoms of an obstructed airway.

3-4. Place the steps of performing a needle and surgical cricothyroidotomy in the correct order of performance.

SUGGESTION After completing the assignment, complete the exercises of this lesson. These exercises will help you to achieve the lesson objectives.

LESSON 3

CRICOTHYROIDOTOMY

Section I. GENERAL CONSIDERATIONS

3-1. DEFINITION

A cricothyroidotomy is an emergency surgical procedure to provide a temporary airway between the cricoid cartilage and thyroid cartilage because there is a total obstruction in the normal oropharyngeal air-exchange route. The cricothyroidotomy site consists of the larynx, which contains the thyroid cartilage (Adam's apple); the cricoid cartilage; the cricothyroid membrane (between the cartilages); the thyroid gland; and the vocal cords. In a needle cricothyroidotomy or a surgical cricothyroidotomy, the cricothyroid membrane is penetrated. Figure 3-1 shows the location of the cricothyroid membrane.

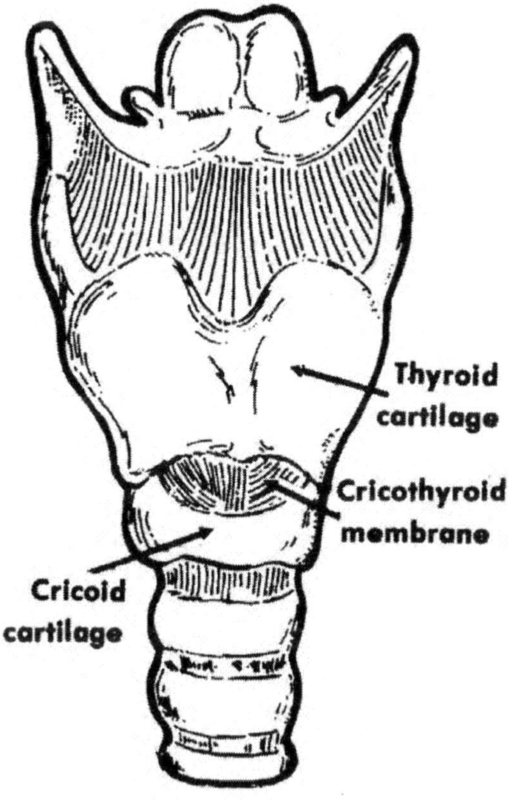

Figure 3-1. Location of the cricothyroid membrane.

3-2. CONDITIONS REQUIRING CRICOTHYROIDOTOMY

a. **Trauma to the Larynx.** A blow to the larynx with a blunt instrument can cause destruction of the structure that supports the larynx. This allows the airway to collapse during inspiration (breathing in) and to close. A blow to the larynx with a blunt object may cause severe swelling (edema). This swelling may not occur for up to 48 hours following the injury, and the swelling may result in the airway being closed. Monitor a casualty with possible or suspected injury to the larynx constantly during the period immediately following such an injury.

b. **Foreign Bodies/Objects.** Foreign bodies such as dislocated teeth or dentures or accumulations of blood, mucus, or vomitus. Foreign objects, accidentally ingested and obstructing the airway, may be the greatest cause of upper airway obstruction. In very young children, foreign objects in the airway may be the result of not knowing how to chew and swallow properly or an underdeveloped epiglottal reflex. In adults airway obstruction is frequently associated with eating coarse meats and vegetables. Airway obstruction in adults is often misdiagnosed as a heart attack (cafe coronary), but the person is really suffering from something obstructing the airway.

c. **Soft Tissue Involvement.** Soft tissue involvement may cause swelling which results in the airway being obstructed. Possible reasons for the swelling include an anaphylactic reaction or flash burns involving trauma to the larynx.

3-3. TYPES/COMPLICATIONS

a. **Types.** There are two types of cricothyroidotomy: needle cricothyroidotomy (also called percutaneous transtracheal ventilation) and surgical cricothyroidotomy.

b. **Complications.** Although a cricothyroidotomy is a relatively safe procedure, complications can occur. Bleeding is the most common complication, but it is usually minor and controllable. False passage is another complication: that is, accidentally entering a passage other than the airway. Complications also include damage to the vocal cords and larynx (if the incision is made incorrectly), mediastinal emphysema, subcutaneous emphysems, and infection.

CAUTION: Resuscitation techniques may be necessary. In such a case, use a bag-valve--mask, demand valve resuscitator, and suction device.

3-4. SIGNS/SYMPTOMS OF AN OBSTRUCTED AIRWAY

The absence of respiration, universal choking sign, and inability to speak are all signs/symptoms of an obstructed airway. On looking at the casualty, you may see that his chest is fully expanded with the rib margins being prominent while the intercostal spaces are depressed. Another sign is slightly bluish discoloration of the skin and mucous membrane because of oxygen deficiency (cyanosis).

Section II. NEEDLE CRICOTHYROIDOTOMY

3-5. EQUIPMENT

To perform a needle cricothyroidotomy, you will need this equipment: iodine preparation kit, large bore needles (12-gauge or 14-gauge), cannula-over-needle device (optional), and tape.

3-6. PROCEDURE

This procedure must be done within four minutes.

a. Place the casualty in the supine position.

b. Extend the casualty's neck by placing a large, rolled-up towel or pillow under his neck or between his shoulder blades so that the airway is straight. Prep the area with povidine-iodine.

c. If you suspect that the casualty has a cervical (neck) injury, DO NOT extend the neck.

d. Palpate the thyroid notch and the cricoid cartilage and locate the cricothyroid membrane.

e. Stabilize the larynx between the thumb and the index and middle fingers of one hand and firmly insert the needle perpendicularly into the membrane.

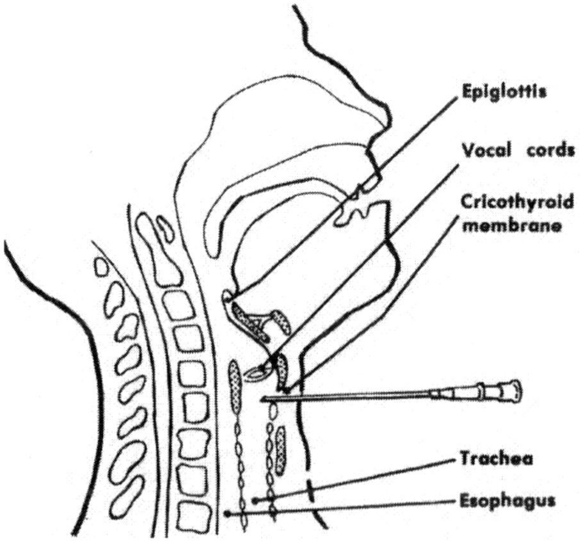

Figure 3-2. Inserting the needle perpendicularly into the cricothyroid membrane.

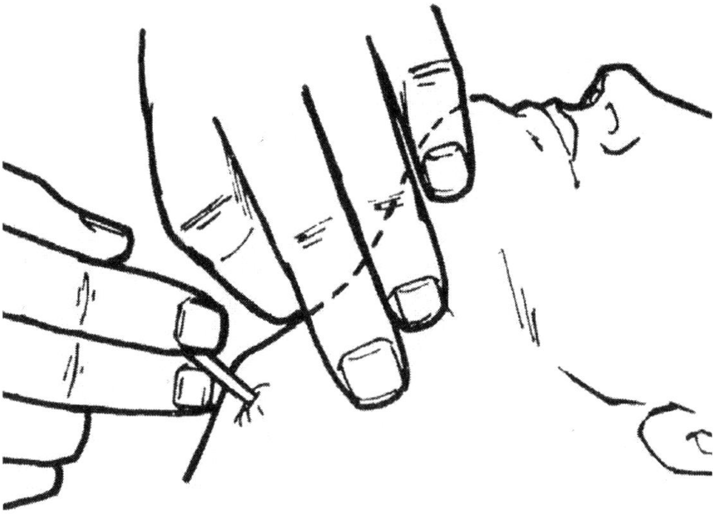

Figure 3-3. Inserting the needle.

f. As the larynx is entered, air will pass back and forth through the needle with the patient's respiratory activity.

g. When the needle is inside the larynx, direct it downward and toward the back (posteriorly) to avoid penetrating the esophagus. Insert an additional needle if the airway you have formed is not sufficient.

CAUTION: This procedure is more risky on a casualty with a tendency to bleed readily or with a large, thick neck. It may be difficult to locate the cricothyroid membrane on a person with a thick neck. If you feel resistance when the needle passes through the cricothyroid membrane, the needle has penetrated the other side of the tracheal cartilage.

h. Stabilize the needle with adhesive tape. Wrap a 6-inch to 8-inch strip of tape around the needles once at the place where the needles exit the skin. Press the ends of the tape around the needles so the needles are held in place and do not come off.

i. Keep the casualty's head relatively immobile.

j. Make preparations for a more permanent airway control. Use an endotracheal intubation or tracheostomy if the airway needs to be artificially maintained for a prolonged time.

k. The procedure may be varied by using a cannula-over-needle device. To do this, remove the needle and allow the catheter to remain in place after it is positioned.

Section III. SURGICAL CRICOTHYROIDOTOMY

3-7. GENERAL

A surgical cricothyroidotomy is the first treatment action when the airway is obstructed by swelling associated with burns, anaphylactic reaction, edema, or a crushing injury to the larynx. IT IS THE LAST RESORT FOR ALL OTHER TYPES OF OBSTRUCTION. This task should NOT be performed on infants and children. Only casualties with a total upper airway obstruction or casualties with inhalation burns should be considered for surgical cricothyroidotomy.

3-8. EQUIPMENT

To perform surgical cricothyroidotomy, you will need the following equipment:

a. Any cutting instrument:

(1) Scissors.

(2) Pocket knife.

(3) Tin can (edge).

(4) Scalpel.

b. If a dilator (an instrument used for stretching an opening) is not available, you may use one of the following to enlarge the opening:

(1) Hemostats (small surgical clamp for constricting a blood vessel).

(2) Needle holders.

(3) Small retractors (Weitlaner).

(4) Knife handle.

(5) Pair of keys.

(6) Cannula (noncollapsible tube to maintain airway).

c. Tape or something to hold the tube in place.

3-9. PROCEDURE

This procedure must be performed within 4 minutes.

a. Place the casualty in the supine position with the neck straight and slightly hyperextended. If you suspect that a casualty has a cervical injury, do not hyperextend the neck. Place a large, rolled-up towel under the casualty's neck or between the shoulder blades so the airway is straight.

b. Locate the cricothyroid space. To do this, palpate the thyroid cartilage (Adam's Apple) with the index finger of one hand. Slide the finger down until you feel the cricothyroid space. (The cricoid cartilage is next).

c. Move the finger upward to the cricothyroid space and cleanse the area. (Cleansing the area may not be possible in a field situation.)

d. Raise a tent of skin overlying the cricothyroid space, using your index finger and thumb.

e. With the cutting instrument in your other hand, make a one and one-half inch horizontal incision through the tented skin down to the cricothyroid space.

f. Reidentify the cricothyroid space by touch and sight.

g. Stabilize the larynx with one hand and make a 1 1/2-inch horizontal incision through the elastic tissues of the cricothyroid membrane.

h. Insert the dilator through the opening.

i. Separate the blades of the dilator to make a larger opening. A rush of air through the opening may be noted.

j. Insert the end of the cannula between the blades of the dilator. The cannula should be in the trachea and directed toward the lungs.

k. Secure the cannula in place to reduce the movement in the opening and to keep the casualty from inhaling the cannula. You may perform mouth to cannula resuscitation if necessary. Inserting the cannula may stimulate reflex coughing. This may aid in clearing the airway, but it is still important to secure the cannula properly.

l. Suction this way. Insert the suction catheter 4 to 5 inches into the cannula. Then, apply suction only when you are withdrawing the catheter. One cc of saline solution may be introduced in the airway to loosen secretions and make suctioning easier. Always allow the casualty to take breaths between efforts to suction.

m. Make a y-shaped cut in a 4" by 4" gauze pad. Place it under the edge of the cannula to prevent irritation to the casualty. (Fold the pad when placing it under the cannula; do not cut the pad at this point.)

n. Place a saline-moistened 4" by 4" gauze pad over the cannula opening to provide moisture in the airway.

Continue with Exercises

EXERCISES, LESSON 3

INSTRUCTIONS. Answer the following exercises by writing the answer in the space provided or by selecting the lettered response that best meets the requirement of the exercise .

After you have completed all of these exercises, turn to "Solutions to Exercises" at the end of the lesson and check your answers. For each exercise answered incorrectly, reread the material referenced with the solution.

1. A cricothyroidotomy can provide a temporary airway between the

   ________________and the ________________when there is a total airway obstruction.

2. List the five parts of the cricothyroidotomy site.

   a. ____.

   b. ____.

   c. ____.

   d. ____.

3. List three reasons a person might need a cricothyroidotomy.

   a. ____.

   b. ____.

   c. ____.

4. Signs and symptoms of an obstructed airway include absence of ____________,

   universal __________________________ signs, and inability to _____________.

5. Although a cricothyroidotomy is a relatively safe procedure, complications include bleeding, entering a passage other than the airway, and damaging

   the_________________________ and the larynx.

6. The correct position of the casualty is the ______________________ position when you are going to perform a needle cricothyroidotomy.

7. There is a greater risk when performing a cricothyroidotomy on a person with a large thick neck because of ______________________________.

8. In the procedure of surgical cricothyroidotomy, a dilator is used to __________.

9. In a surgical cricothyroidotomy, the incision made is _______________ long.

10. These are the beginning steps in the procedure of performing a needle cricothyroidotomy. The steps are not in the order in which you would do them. Choose the response which lists the steps in the correct order of performance.

    1. Raise a tent of skin overlying the cricothyroid space.
    2. Pace the casualty in the correct position.
    3. Locate the cricothyroid space.
    4. Make a horizontal incision cutting down to the cricothyroid space.
    5. Move a finger upward to the cricothyroid space and cleanse the area.

    a. 3,2,1,5,4.

    b. 4,1,3,2,5.

    c. 1,4,2,3,5.

    d. 1,3,5,1,4.

11. These are steps in the procedure of performing a surgical cricothyroidotomy. The steps are not in the order in which you would do them. Choose the response which lists the steps in the correct order of performance.

1. Stabilize the larynx with one hand and make a 1/2 inch horizontal incision through the elastic tissues of the cricothyroid membrane.

2. Insert the cannula end between the blades of the dilator.

3. Insert the dilator, separating its blades to make a larger opening.

4. Reidentify the cricothyroid space.

5. Secure the cannula in place.

a. 1,4,3,2,5.

b. 4,1,3,2,5.

c. 1,4,2,3,5

d. 1,3,5,1,4.

Check Your Answers on Next Page

SOLUTIONS TO EXERCISES, LESSON 3

1. Cricoid cartilage, thyroid cartilage. (para 3-1)

2. Thyroid cartilage.
   Cricoid cartilage.
   Cricothyroid membrane.
   Thyroid gland.
   Vocal cords. (para 3-1)

3. Trauma to the larynx.
   Foreign bodies/objects obstructing the airway.
   Soft tissue involvement (swelling) obstructing the airway. (paras 3-2a, 2b)

4. Respiration, choking, speak at all. (para 3-4)

5. Vocal cords. (para 3-3b)

6. Supine. (para 3-6a)

7. It is difficult to locate the cricothyroid membrane. (para 3-6g CAUTION)

8. Stretch the opening after the incision through the cricothyroid membrane is made. (para 3-8b)

9. 1 1/2 inches. (para 3-9g)

10. c. (para 3-9a through 9e)

11. b. (para 3-9f through 9k)

End of Lesson 3

Cardiac Impairment

Subcourse MD0571

This page intentionally left blank.

U.S. ARMY MEDICAL DEPARTMENT CENTER AND SCHOOL
FORT SAM HOUSTON, TEXAS 78234-6100

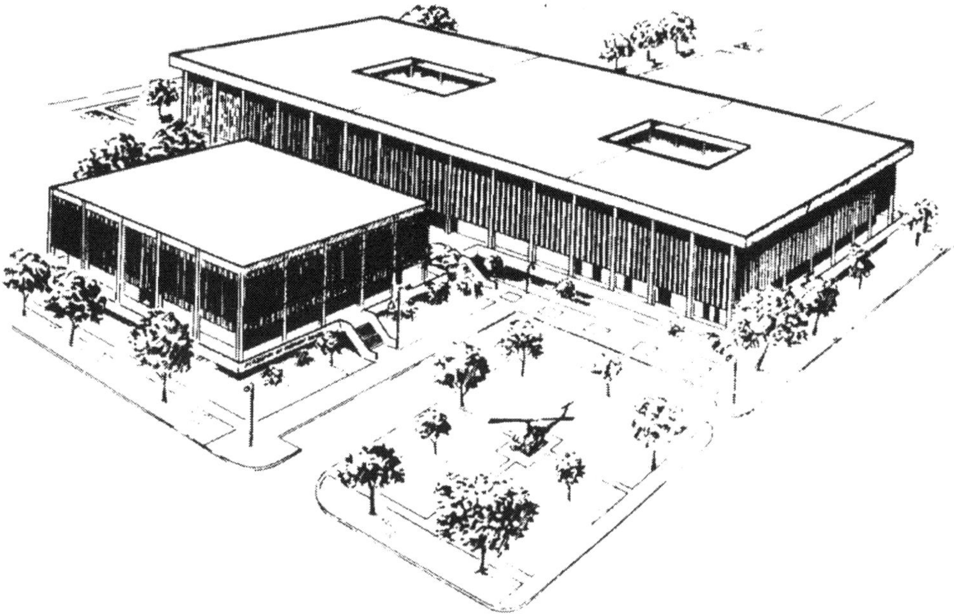

CARDIAC IMPAIRMENT

SUBCOURSE MD0571 EDITION 100

DEVELOPMENT

This subcourse is approved for resident and correspondence course instruction. It reflects the current thought of the Academy of Health Sciences and conforms to printed Department of the Army doctrine as closely as currently possible. Development and progress render such doctrine continuously subject to change.

ADMINISTRATION

For comments or questions regarding enrollment, student records, or shipments, contact the Nonresident Instruction Branch at DSN 471-5877, commercial (210) 221-5877, toll-free 1-800-344-2380; fax: 210-221-4012 or DSN 471-4012, e-mail accp@amedd.army.mil, or write to:

COMMANDER
AMEDDC&S
ATTN MCCS HSN
2105 11TH STREET SUITE 4192
FORT SAM HOUSTON TX 78234-5064

Approved students whose enrollments remain in good standing may apply to the Nonresident Instruction Branch for subsequent courses by telephone, letter, or e-mail.

Be sure your social security number is on all correspondence sent to the Academy of Health Sciences.

CLARIFICATION OF TRAINING LITERATURE TERMINOLOGY

When used in this publication, words such as "he," "him," "his," and "men" are intended to include both the masculine and feminine genders, unless specifically stated otherwise or when obvious in context.

TABLE OF CONTENTS

Lesson Paragraphs

INTRODUCTION

1 BASIC CARDIAC LIFE SUPPORT

Section I. General Information 1-1--1-7
Section II. Rescue Breathing 1-8--1-9
Section III. Chest Compressions 1-10--1-12
Section IV. One-Rescuer Method CPR 1-13--1-14
Section V. Two-Rescuer Method CPR 1-15--1-20
Section VI. CPR Complications/CPR Termination 1-21--1-22
Exercises

2 DYSRHYTHMIA RECOGNITION AND TREATMENT

Section I. Dysrhythmia 2-1--2-2
Section II. Electrophysiology 2-3--2-5
Section III. Rhythms/Heart Blocks 2-6--2-12
Exercises

3 CARDIAC ARREST (DEFIBRILLATION)

Section I. Review of the Cardiovascular System and the Respiratory System 3-1--3-5
Section II. General Considerations Regarding Cardiac Arrest 3-6--3-10
Section III. Major Management Techniques of Cardiac Arrest 3-11--3-12
Section IV. Cardioversion 3-15--3-18

CORRESPONDENCE COURSE OF
THE ACADEMY OF HEALTH SCIENCES, UNITED STATES ARMY

SUBCOURSE MD0571

CARDIAC IMPAIRMENT

INTRODUCTION

In this subcourse, you will study cardiac arrest; basic life support, to include rescue breathing; chest compressions; and recognition and treatment of cardiac dysrhythmias. This information will aid you in maintaining and improving the health of soldiers. In that pursuit, do your best to achieve the objectives of this subcourse.

Subcourse Components:

This subcourse consists of three lessons:

Lesson 1 Basic Cardiac Life Support.
Lesson 2 Dysrhythmia Recognition and Treatment.
Lesson 3 Cardiac Arrest.

Study Suggestions:

Here are some suggestions that may be helpful to you in completing this subcourse:

--Read and study each lesson carefully.
--Complete the subcourse lesson by lesson. After completing each lesson, work the exercises at the end of the lesson, marking your answers in this booklet.

--After completing each set of lesson exercises, compare your answers with those on the solution sheet that follows the exercises. If you have answered an exercise incorrectly, check the reference cited after the answer on the solution sheet to determine why your response was not the correct one.

Credit Awarded:

To receive credit hours, you must be officially enrolled and complete an examination furnished by the Nonresident Instruction Branch at Fort Sam Houston, Texas. Upon successful completion of the examination for this subcourse, you will be awarded 8 credit hours.

You can enroll by going to the web site http://atrrs.army.mil and enrolling under "Self Development" (School Code 555).

A listing of correspondence courses and subcourses available through the Nonresident Instruction Section is found in Chapter 4 of DA Pamphlet 350-59, Army Correspondence Course Program Catalog. The DA PAM is available at the following website: http://www.usapa.army.mil/pdffiles/p350-59.pdf.

LESSON ASSIGNMENT

LESSON 1 Basic Cardiac Life Support.

LESSON ASSIGNMENT Paragraphs 1-1 through 1-22.

LESSON OBJECTIVES After completing this lesson, you should be able to:

1-1. Identify the steps in performing one-rescuer CARDIOPULMONARY RESUSCITATION (CPR).

1-2. Identify the steps in performing two-rescuer CPR.

1-3. Identify the steps in switching from one-rescuer CPR to two-rescuer CPR.

1-4. Identify the steps in switching positions with another rescuer while you are both performing two-rescuer CPR.

SUGGESTION After completing the assignment, complete the exercises of this lesson. These exercises will help you to achieve the lesson objectives.

LESSON 1

CARDIAC IMPAIRMENT

Section I. GENERAL INFORMATION

1-1. INTRODUCTION TO CARDIOPULMONARY RESUSCITATION

Blood supplies the cells of the body with oxygen. In an emergency, you must ensure that this supply of oxygen continues. The supply of oxygen to the body cells is threatened whenever the person stops breathing on his own, or when the person's heart stops pumping blood. When the oxygen supply fails, cells begin to die. The length of time required for a cell to die after the oxygen supply has stopped depends upon several factors. One of the most important factors is the type of cell involved. Brain cells are the most sensitive. Permanent brain damage usually occurs if the oxygen supply is stopped for more than 4 minutes. The following sections deal with restoring the breathing process to a person who has stopped breathing for himself and restoring the heartbeat to a person who heart has stopped beating. The combination of techniques that provides basic emergency life support by keeping oxygenated blood flowing in the brain during such occurrences is called cardiopulmonary resuscitation (CPR).

1-2. SUDDEN DEATH

Sudden death is defined as the unexpected cessation of respiration and functional circulation. There are two stages of sudden death: clinical death and biological death.

a. **Clinical Deaths.** Clinical death means that the heartbeat and breathing have stopped. This condition is reversible. Sudden death is abrupt and unexpected clinical death.

b. **Biological Death.** Biological death is permanent cellular damage due to lack of oxygen. The brain cells are the most sensitive to lack of oxygen. Irreversible brain damage occurs within 4 to 6 minutes. Biological death is a final condition.

c. **Difference Between Clinical Death and Biological Death.** Clinical death occurs as soon as the heart stops beating and the person stops breathing. Clinical death results in unconsciousness. This condition can be reversed by cardiopulmonary resuscitation. If CPR is not initiated, biological death usually occurs 4 to 6 minutes after clinical death. Biological death involves irreversible brain damage.

1-3. RECOVERY PROBABILITY RATES

If basic life support (BLS) is delayed from 1 to 4 minutes after cardiac arrest, the recovery rate is 50 percent. If BLS is delayed 7 minutes after cardiac arrest, the recovery rate is 8 percent. If BLS is delayed for 10 minutes after cardiac arrest, the recovery rate is less than one percent.

1-4. COMMON CAUSES OF SUDDEN DEATH

Listed below are the common causes of sudden death:

a. Drowning.

b. Electrical shock.

c. Poisoning.

d. Suffocation.

e. Smoke inhalation.

f. Choking on food or other objects.

g. Sensitivity reaction and anaphylactic shock.

h. Automobile accident.

i. Medical reasons.

j. Myocardial infarction.

1-5. RESCUER RESPONSIBILITIES DURING CARDIOPULMONARY RESUSCITATION

A person performing CPR has two basic responsibilities: prevent biological death of the casualty and get competent help. To prevent biological death, you must be able to recognize the nature of the emergency. You must also be able to provide artificial breathing and artificial circulation <u>immediately</u>. The ability to get competent help involves knowing the civilian telephone numbers for emergencies (911 in major metropolitan areas) including special numbers on a military installation including the general emergency number, the fire department number, and military police, number.

1-6. DEFINITION OF CARDIOPULMONARY RESUSCITATION

The term "cardio-" refers to the heart; the term "pulmonary-" refers to the lungs; and the term "resuscitation" means to bring a person who appears to be dead to consciousness. Thus, cardiopulmonary resuscitation means restoring lung function (breathing) and heart function (blood circulation) to a person who is clinically dead. Cardiopulmonary resuscitation is usually referred to simply as CPR. Cardiopulmonary resuscitation is composed of an assessment (evaluation) phase during which the responsiveness of the person is determined followed by the three basic maneuvers: opening the airway, rescue breathing, and chest compressions.

1-7. IMPORTANCE OF CARDIOPULMONARY RESUSCITATION

Past experience with situations requiring basic life support measures (restoring breathing and heartbeat) has demonstrated that a significant number of casualties can be successfully resuscitated if CPR is provided <u>promptly</u> and followed by more advanced cardiac life support. Prompt response is critical. The American Heart Association reports that the longer CPR is delayed, the lower the survival rate.

SECTION II. RESCUE BREATHING

1-8. INTRODUCTION

A person who is not breathing will die in a short time because the cells are not receiving a fresh supply of oxygen. Cardiopulmonary resuscitation, in this case, one-rescuer CPR, is a method by which the rescuer forces air into the casualty's lungs. The casualty's blood can then pick up oxygen from the air that has been forced into his lungs. Even though the air comes from the rescuer, it still contains plenty of oxygen. When the rescuer stops blowing air through the casualty's mouth (or nose) and breaks the seal over the casualty's mouth (or nose), the casualty's body will exhale without assistance from the rescuer. Thus, CPR acts as a substitute for the normal inhaling and exhaling process.

1-9. RESCUE BREATHING PROCEDURE

a. **Evaluation (Assessment) Phase.** If you see someone lying on the ground not moving, evaluate the situation first. Part of this evaluation is simply observing the surroundings. Does it appear that the person could have been injured in a traffic accident, by a fall, or by some other violent accident? If any of these accidents could have occurred, consider that the casualty could have a spinal fracture and take some special precautions if you must perform CPR. If you cannot see any evidence of an accident, the casualty may have suffered a heart attack without a spinal injury. Another part of the evaluation is a quick check to see if the person really is unconscious. Tap the casualty on the shoulder. Shake him gently (take care not to cause additional injury), and shout, "Are you O.K.?" (**NOTE**: Do not shake the casualty if you suspect spinal injury--just shout. Even if you do not suspect spinal damage, do not shake the person in a violent manner. Violent shaking could aggravate other injuries the casualty may have suffered.) If the casualty responds (conscious), give whatever aid is needed. If he does not respond (unconscious), conscious), continue with your rescue efforts. It will take from four to ten seconds to establish unconsciousness. Whether the casualty is conscious or unconscious, call for additional help, if such help is available.

b. **Positioning the Casualty.** You must position a casualty flat on his back before beginning CPR. If the casualty is lying in a supine position (on his back), place his arms at his side and proceed to establish an open airway (para 1-9c). If the casualty is in a prone position (on his chest), turn him onto his back using the procedures given below and shown in figure 2-1. These procedures allow the casualty's body to be turned as a unit and minimize the likelihood that injuries will be aggravated. It is especially important to use these procedures if you suspect that the casualty may have an injury to his spine. Follow this procedure:

(1) Straighten the casualty's legs (figure 1-1 A).

(2) Take the casualty's arm that is nearest to you and move it so that it is straight and above his head (figure 1-1 A). Then, move his other arm so that it is straight and above his head also.

(3) Kneel beside the casualty. Your knees should be near his chest area, but there should be enough space between you and the casualty for you to roll him onto his back (figure 1-1 A).

(4) Support the casualty's head and neck by placing your hand that is nearest his head on the back of his head and neck (figure 1-1 A).

(5) With your other hand, grasp the casualty under his far arm (figure 1-1 B).

(6) Roll the casualty towards you (figure 1-1 B). Use a steady and even pull, turning the casualty's body as a unit so that his head and neck stay in line with his back.

(7) Return the casualty's arms to his side (figure 1-1C). If his legs are crossed, straighten them so that they are not crossed.

NOTE: Be sure that the casualty is on a hard surface. A firm surface is necessary for chest compressions to be effective. Appropriate surfaces include the ground, a backboard, and a bed board.

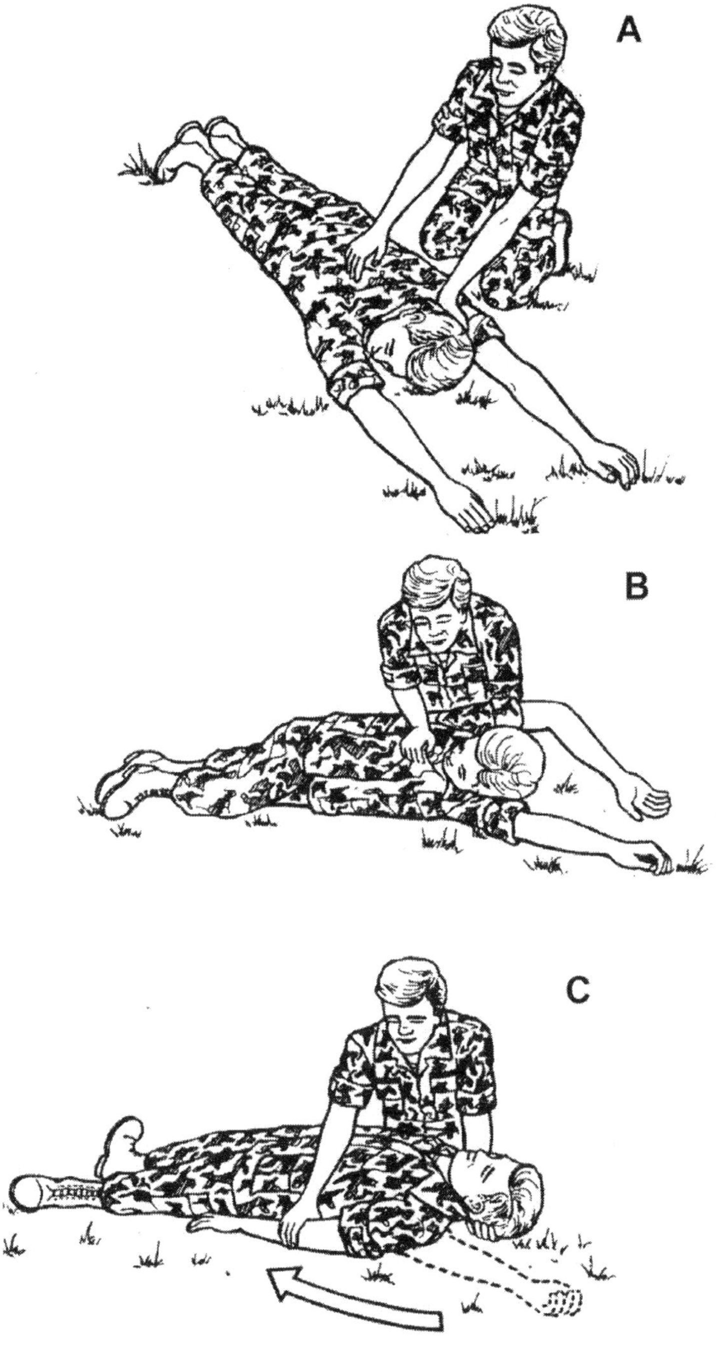

Figure 1-1. Rolling a casualty onto his back.

c. **Establishing an Airway.** Sometimes an unconscious casualty who is breathing poorly will resume normal breathing when his head is positioned so that his airway is reopened. This is especially true when the casualty's tongue has caused the airway to become blocked. Since the tongue is attached to the lower jaw, repositioning the jaw forward can lift the tongue away from the back of the throat and reopen the airway. Two commonly used methods of establishing an airway are the head-tilt/chin-lift method and the jaw-thrust method. Establishing an airway should take between 3 and 5 seconds.

(1) Head-tilt/chin-lift method. This is the preferred method of opening the casualty's airway if a spinal fracture in the neck region is not suspected. In addition, loose dentures can be handled easier using the head-tilt/chin-lift method than when using another method. Procedures for the head-tilt/chin-lift method of establishing an airway are given here:

(a) Kneel at the side of the casualty's head.

(b) Place the fingertips of one hand under the bony part of his chin.

(c) Place your other hand on his forehead.

(d) Press on his forehead to make the head tilt back while lifting his chin forward (figure 1-2 A). Lift until the teeth are almost brought together. The mouth should not be closed as this could prevent air from entering the casualty's airway. The thumb is usually not used in lifting the chin. In some cases, the thumb may be used to depress the casualty's lower lip slightly to keep his mouth open.

(2) Jaw-thrust method. The jaw-thrust method is an effective method to use in opening the airway. The procedure is as follows:

(a) Kneel beside the casualty.

(b) Rest your elbows on the same surface on which the casualty is lying.

(c) Place your hands on either side of the casualty's head. Grasp the angles of the casualty's lower jaw.

(d) Lift the casualty's lower jaw forward and tilt his head backward at the same time (figure 1-2 B).

(e) If you must perform rescue breathing, pull the casualty's lower lip open with your thumb and close the casualty's nostrils by placing your cheek tightly against his nostrils.

NOTE: This technique is very successful in opening the airway, but it is tiring to the rescuer and difficult to perform.

CAUTION: If you think the casualty has a neck injury, use the jaw-thrust method without the head-lift. If the jaw-thrust method does not open the airway, then use the head-tilt method.

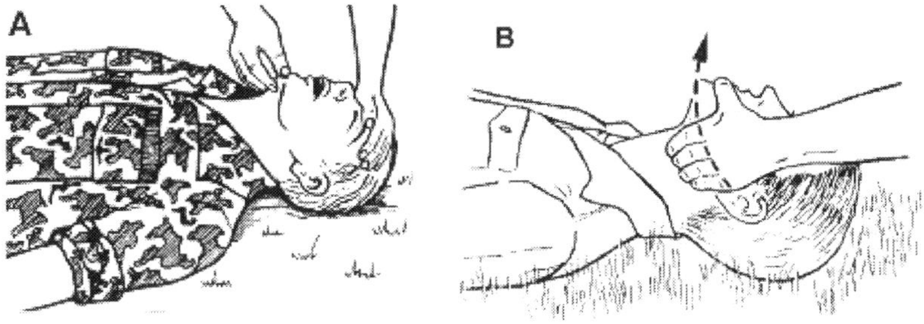

Figure 1-2. Establishing an airway A Head-tilt/chin-lift method. B Jaw-thrust method.

d. **Checking for Breathing.** Check to see if the casualty is breathing. Many times, opening the airway is all that is needed to restore breathing in an unconscious person. While you are doing the check, maintain the casualty's airway using the head-tilt/chin-lift or the jaw-thrust method.

NOTE: This is the first time you actually check to see if the casualty is breathing. Even if an unconscious casualty is breathing when you find him, his breathing could deteriorate or stop altogether while you are performing other measures. That is why you must take the precaution of positioning the casualty and establishing an airway.

(1) Place your ear over the casualty's mouth and nose and look towards the casualty's chest (figure 1-3). For the best results, your ear should be touching his nose.

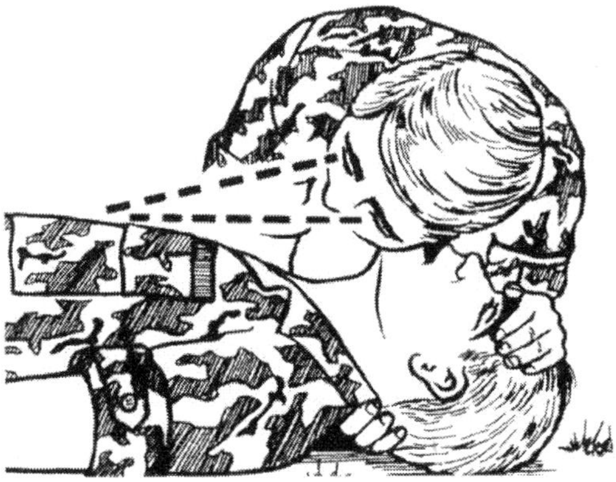

Figure 1-3. Checking a casualty for breathing by the head-tilt/chin-lift method.

(2) Look at the casualty's at the casualty's chest. If the casualty is breathing, you should be able to see the chest rise and fall.

(3) Listen for the sound of breathing (air being inhaled and exhaled).

(4) Feel for the flow of air on the side of your face, the air flow being caused by the casualty exhaling.

e. **Evaluating Your Findings.**

(1) If your check shows that the casualty is breathing, take measures to maintain his airway.

(2) If your check shows that the casualty is not breathing, reposition his head and neck (para 1-7b) and check for breathing a second time. If he is still not breathing, you must perform CPR immediately.

f. **Rescue Breathing.** Forcing an unconscious casualty to inhale and exhale is the part of CPR termed "rescue breathing" or "ventilating the casualty." (Ventilation simply means that you are supplying the casualty's lungs with fresh air.) There are three methods of rescue breathing. Mouth-to-mouth is the method normally used. Mouth-to-nose, an alternate method, is used when the casualty's mouth cannot be opened or when you are unable to achieve a tight seal around the casualty's mouth. Procedures for performing mouth-to-nose rescue breathing are given in paragraph f (2) below.

NOTE: If the casualty has had his larynx removed surgically, there will be an opening in the neck for breathing purposes. This opening, called a stoma, can be used to perform mouth-to-stoma rescue breathing.

(1) Mouth-to-mouth rescue breathing. Perform mouth-to-mouth ventilations in the following manner:

(a) Gently pinch the casualty's nose closed. The casualty's nostrils must be closed so that air will not escape when you blow air into his mouth. Using the thumb and index finger of your hand on the casualty's forehead, pinch his nostrils closed gently (figure 1-4). Keep the heel of your hand on the casualty's forehead and maintain enough pressure to maintain the head-tilt. Your other hand should stay on the casualty's chin or neck so the airway remains open.

(b) Give two full breaths within 3 seconds.

NOTE: This is a change. Previously, the directions were to give "four quick breaths." It is believed those breaths put too much air in the lungs and caused complications such as gastric distention.

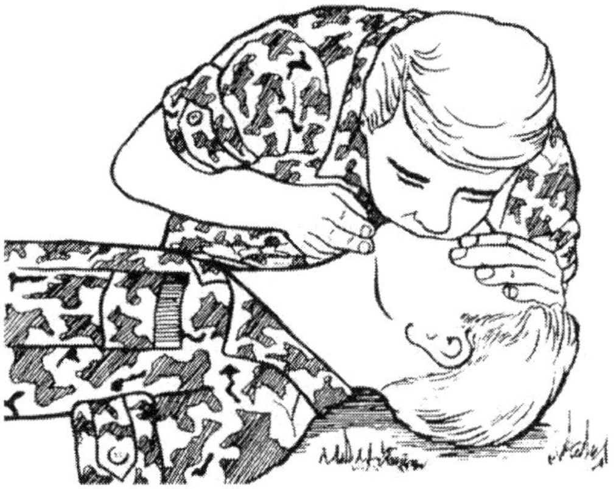

Figure 1-4. Administering mouth-to-mouth rescue breathing by the head-tilt/chin-lift.

1 Take a deep breath.

2 Seal your lips around the outside of the casualty's mouth thus creating an airtight seal.

3 Blow two full breaths within three seconds into the casualty's mouth.

4 If your initial attempt to ventilate the casualty is unsuccessful, reposition the casualty's head and repeat rescue breathing.

5 After the second breath, break the seal over the casualty's mouth and release his nose. The casualty's body will exhale without effort on your part.

6 Check for breathing.

(c) Evaluate the effectiveness of the two breaths.

1 If the casualty's chest did not rise and fall, then fresh air is not getting into his lungs. Try repositioning the casualty's head to open his airway more. If the head-tilt/chin-lift method or the jaw-thrust is being used, lift the chin more. If the head-tilt/neck-lift method is being used, lift the neck more. After you have done this, administer two full breaths within 3 seconds again.

2 If casualty's chest still does not rise even after you have tried to increase the airway opening, the casualty probably has an object blocking his airway. Administer manual thrusts and finger sweeps to open the airway. (Manual thrust = a thrust delivered to the abdomen or breast bone to force air out of the lungs, thus, expelling a foreign body from the airway.)

3 If the casualty begins breathing again on his own, look for injuries. **DO NOT** leave the casualty since his breathing may stop again. The casualty may still require help to keep his airway open.

4 If air goes in and out of the casualty's lungs, but he does not start breathing on his own, administer the rescue breathing procedures given in the paragraphs that follow.

(d) Feel for the carotid pulse. After you have successfully given the initial two full breaths, check the casualty's pulse. Getting fresh air into the casualty's lungs will not help if his heart is not beating and the blood is not circulating. There are two major arteries, called the carotid arteries, in the neck. On the left side of the trachea is one artery (windpipe); the other artery is on the right side of the trachea. Either artery may be used to check the casualty's carotid pulse, but normally you should use the artery on the side of the neck nearest you. The carotid pulse is used because you are already near the neck and a pulse can sometimes be felt at the carotid arteries when the pulse is too weak to be detected at arteries further from the heart. Procedures for checking the casualty's carotid pulse are given below. The procedures take about five seconds. Follow these procedures to feel for the carotid pulse:

1 Place the index and middle fingers of your hand that is not on the casualty's forehead on the side of the casualty's trachea (figure 1-5). Use the side nearest you. (**IMPORTANT:** Do not use your thumb to feel for the pulse. The pulse you find may be your thumb's pulse, not the casualty's carotid pulse.)

2 Slide your finger into the groove beside the Adam's apple (The "Adam's apple" is actually the larynx. The Adam's apple is smaller in females than in males.

3 Gently feel for the pulse. Maintain the head-tilt with your hand on the casualty's forehead.

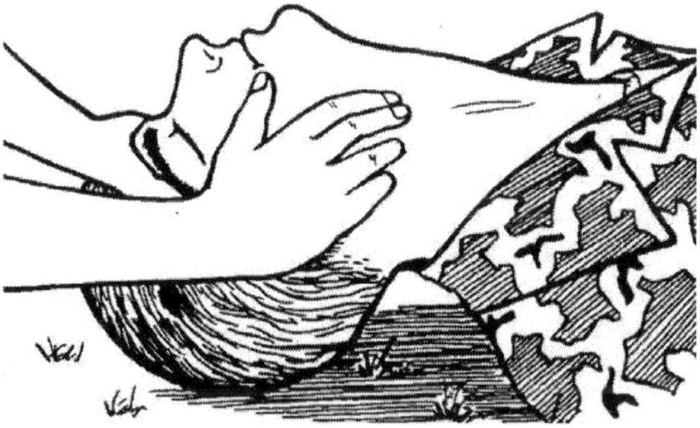

Figure 1-5. Feeling for the casualty's carotid pulse.

4 Send someone to get help.

5 If no pulse is felt, begin CPR immediately. If a pulse can be felt, continue with rescue breathing procedures given in the next paragraph.

(e) Continue rescue breathing. If the casualty's heart is beating and he is not breathing on his own, continue to administer rescue breathing using the procedure given below. Perform ventilations at a rate of one ventilation every 5 seconds (12 ventilations per minute). Continue to keep the casualty's airway open while performing the ventilations, and follow this procedure:

1 Take a deep breath.

2 Pinch the casualty's nostrils closed; use the thumb and index finger of your hand on his forehead to do this.

3 Place your mouth over the casualty's mouth, making sure that a tight seal is formed.

4 Blow into the casualty's mouth. As you blow, observe the casualty's chest. If his chest does not rise, a sufficient amount of air is not getting into his lungs. This may be caused by these factors: inadequate positioning of the casualty's head, chin, or neck; air leaking from the casualty's nose; air leaking from around your mouth; an airway obstruction; or the breath not being delivered with sufficient force. If a problem exists, correct the problem and continue administering ventilations.

5 Remove your mouth from around the casualty's mouth and release his nose. This allows him to exhale. Remember, the casualty's airway must be kept open so that he can exhale.

6 Recheck the casualty's pulse after every 12 breaths (once per minute). If the pulse is absent, begin administering chest compressions at once.

7 Continue administering rescue breathing at the rate of one breath every 5 seconds until the casualty begins breathing on his own, until you are relieved by a qualified person, until you are ordered to stop by a doctor, or until you are too exhausted to continue.

8 If the casualty begins breathing on his own, monitor him in case his breathing stops again.

9 When possible, evacuate the casualty for further evaluation and treatment by a doctor. If the casualty is not breathing on his own, continue administering rescue breathing during the evacuation.

(2) Mouth-to-nose rescue breathing. Use this technique in the following situations: impossible to open the casualty's mouth; casualty's mouth is seriously injured; or difficult to achieve a tight seal on the casualty's mouth. Open the casualty's airway and follow this procedure for mouth-to-nose rescue breathing:

(a) Close the casualty's mouth completely. Use your hand that is not on the casualty's forehead to lift his jaw and close his mouth. It is important that no air escape through the casualty's mouth when you perform ventilations.

(b) Give two quick, full breaths. Take a deep breath, seal your lips around the casualty's nose and blow into his nose. (See figure 1-6.) Be sure the two quick breaths are given with three seconds. Observe the casualty's chest as you administer the two breaths.

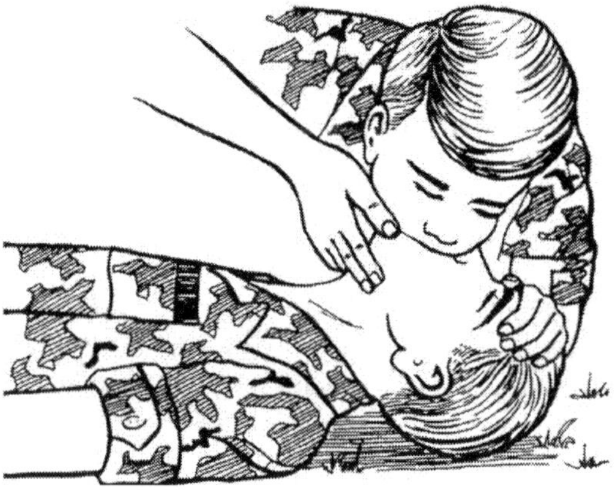

Figure 1-6. Administering mouth-to-nose rescue breathing.

(c) Remove your mouth from the casualty's nose. Either open his mouth or separate his lips so that he can exhale passively.

(d) Evaluate the effectiveness of the two breaths:

1 If the casualty's chest did not rise and fall, try opening his airway more and administer two breaths again. If this does not work, check for an upper airway obstruction and remove any blockage. Then, continue administering breaths until the four quick breaths cause the chest to rise.

2 If the casualty starts to breathe on his own, begin looking for injuries and treat them. Be prepared to resume rescue breathing in case the casualty stops breathing again.

3 If the two breaths caused the casualty's chest to rise and fall but the casualty has not started breathing on-his own, feel for his carotid pulse. If there is no pulse, begin chest compressions as described in Section III of this lesson.

4 If the casualty's heart is still beating and the casualty is not breathing on his own, continue to perform-mouth-to-nose ventilations.

(e) Continue rescue breathing. If the casualty's heart is beating but he is not breathing on his own, perform mouth-to-nose ventilations at a rate of one ventilation every five seconds.

1. Take a deep breath.

2. Close the casualty's mouth.

3. Form a seal over his nose and force air into his nose.

4 Break the seal over the casualty's nose and allow him to exhale (either open his mouth or separate his lips).

5 Check the casualty's pulse after every 12 ventilations. If the pulse is absent, begin administering chest compressions.

6 Continue administering mouth-to-nose ventilations at a rate of 12 ventilations per minute until the casualty is breathing on his own, until you are relieved by a qualified person, until a doctor tells you to stop, or until you are too exhausted to continue rescue breathing.

7 If the casualty begins breathing on his own, monitor him in case his breathing stops again.

8 When possible, evacuate the casualty for further evaluation and treatment by a physician. If the casualty is not breathing on his own, continue administering rescue breathing during the evacuation.

(3) Mouth-to-stoma rescue breathing. Follow the same procedures as for mouth-to-mouth rescue breathing. The difference is that you place your mouth over the neck opening instead of over the mouth, and you hold the mouth closed.

Section III. CHEST COMPRESSIONS

1-10. INTRODUCTION

If the casualty's heart stops beating, the blood stops circulating. When blood stops circulating, cells cannot get oxygen, and they begin to die. The casualty's heart, however, may still be beating even though he has stopped breathing on his own. If his heart stops beating, he will stop breathing also. Just as the rescuer can perform rescue breathing as a substitute for the casualty's normal heartbeat, the rescuer can perform chest compressions to substitute for the casualty's normal heartbeat. In neither case, however, is the substitute measure as efficient as the body's natural process. Cardiopulmonary resuscitation is the combination of rescue breathing and chest compressions.

CARDIOPULMONARY RESUSCITATION = **RESCUE BREATHING** (Substitute for casualty's breathing) + **CHEST COMPRESSIONS** (Substitute for casualty's normal heartbeat)

Figure 1-7. Cardiopulmonary resuscitation.

1-11. EFFECTS OF CHEST COMPRESSIONS

An external chest compression is the application of pressure over the casualty's sternum. External chest compressions force blood to be circulated to the heart, lungs, brain, and other organs. Blood circulated to the lungs by this method plus rescue breathing will maintain a casualty's life until other treatment can be obtained for him. Properly performed external chest compressions alone can produce systolic blood pressure to peak at over 100 mm Hg. The compressions can bring the carotid arterial blood flow up to 35 percent of normal. The heart is located between the sternum and the spine. When the sternum is pressed down far enough into the chest cavity (1 1/2 to 2 inches in an adult), the heart is compressed between the sternum and the spine (figure 1-8 A. When pressure is removed from the sternum, it rises to its normal position. When the sternum rises, the heart resumes its normal shape (figure 1-8 B). Since blood has been forced out of the ventricles during compression, blood flows from the atria into the ventricles as the heart returns to its normal shape. Each pressure-release cycle causes blood to be pumped and is roughly equal to one heartbeat.

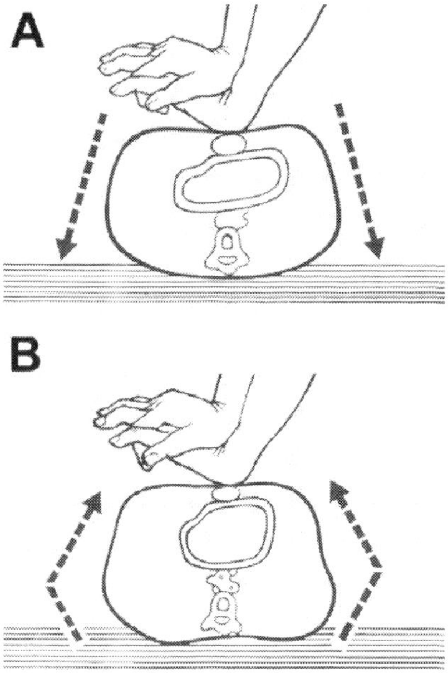

Figure 1-8. Effects of chest compression. A Compression. B Release.

1-12. PROCEDURE FOR CHEST COMPRESSIONS

Be sure the casualty is in the supine position. If the head is elevated above the heart, less or sometimes no blood gets to the brain. If necessary, a board can be placed under the patient's chest to provide a firm, flat surface for the patient to lie on.

a. **Locate the Compression Site.** Determine proper hand position in this manner:

(1) Using the middle and index finger of your hand which is nearest the casualty's legs, find the lower margin of his rib cage on the side of his body closest to you. See figure 1-9 A .

(2) Move your fingers up the casualty's rib cage to the notch where the ribs meet the sternum in the center of the lower part of the chest.

(3) Keep your middle finger on this notch and place your index finger next to the middle finger on the lower end of the sternum. See figure 1-9 B .

(4) Your other hand has been on the casualty's forehead to keep his head in position maintaining the airway. Put the heel of that hand on the lower half of the sternum, close to the index finger that is next to the middle finger in the notch. The thumb side of that hand should be against the index finger of the other hand. The heel is now on the compression site. See figure 1-9 C .

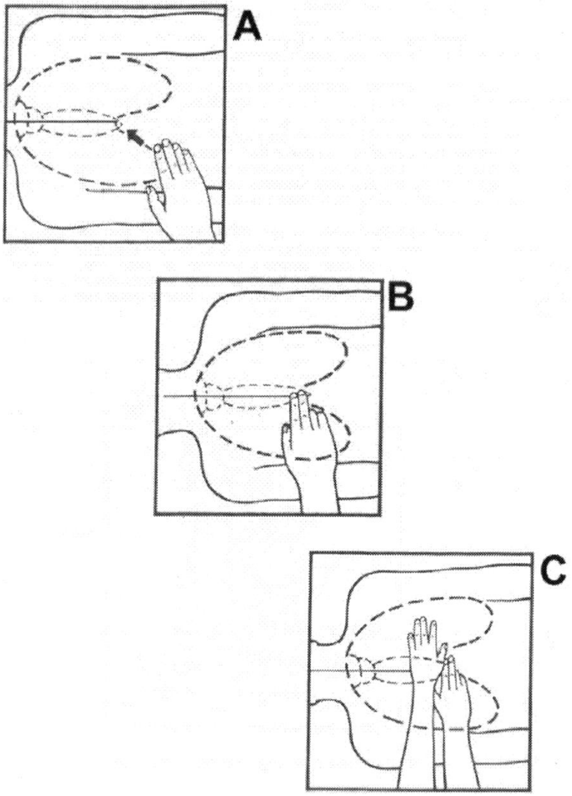

Figure 1-9. Locating the compression site for chest compression.

b. **Position Hands for Giving Chest Compressions.** Follow these steps:

(1) Remove your hand from the notch and put it on top of the hand on the sternum.

(2) Be sure both hands point away from the rescuer (toward the opposite side of the casualty). You may hold your fingers straight or interlocked. You will exert pressure with the HEEL of your hands; therefore, be sure your fingers and palms DO NOT touch the casualty's chest. (See figure 1-10.)

NOTE: An alternate method to this hand position is to grasp the wrist of your hand on the casualty's chest with your hand that had located the lower end of the sternum.

c. **Administer External Chest Compressions.** Proceed in this way:

(1) Lock your elbows with your arms straight. This makes chest compressions more efficient and saves the rescuer's energy.

(2) Position your shoulders directly over your hands so that the thrust for each chest compression is straight down. The casualty's torso may roll if you push other than straight down. If the casualty rolls, the thrust of the chest compression will be much weaker and less effective. Also, the rolling motion of the casualty can make the rescuer very tired and cause additional injury to the casualty. Possible injuries include fractured ribs, fractured xyphoid process, and lacerations (rips or punctures) of internal organs caused by sharp pieces of broken bone.

(3) Push straight down on the sternum so that it goes down 1 1/2 to 2 inches for the normal sized adult. Use your weight when pushing down. Instead of pushing down using your arm and shoulder muscles only, let the weight of your body move forward and use that force to help depress the sternum. Remember to keep your arms straight and your elbows locked during the push. (See figure 1-10.)

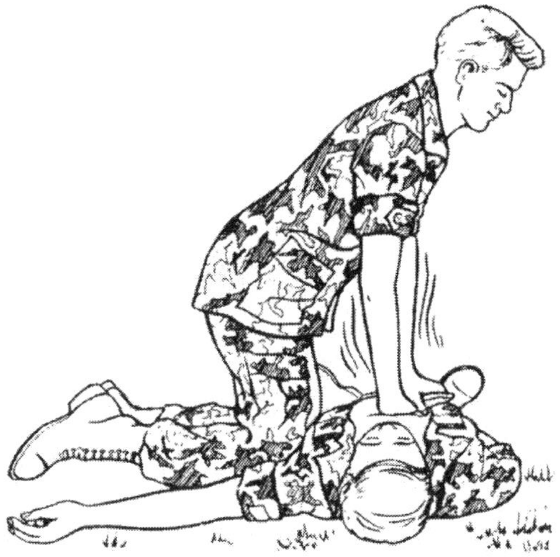

Figure 1-10. Rescuer administering external chest compressions.

(4) Give 15 compressions (10-12 seconds). A compression cycle consists of a thrust which compresses the heart and a release which allows the heart to refill with blood. These compressions are delivered at a rate of 80 cycles per minute (about 11 seconds for each 15 compressions). Delivering chest compressions at this rate will allow the rescuer to administer a total of 60 compressions per minute since some time will be required to administer two breaths after every 15 compressions.

d. **Relax and Allow the Chest to Rise Completely.** Releasing the pressure allows the heart to refill with blood. Release the pressure completely so that the sternum resumes its normal position, but do not remove the heel of your hand from the compression site. If you do lose the compression site, repeat the procedures for finding the site.

e. **Repeat Until 15 Push-Relax Cycles Have Been Completed.** (If One--Rescuer CPR is Being Performed) or five Push-Relax Cycles Have Been Completed (If Two-Rescuer CPR is Being Performed). Establish a definite rhythm and compress at the rate of 80 cycles per minute (15 compressions in 10-12 seconds). Spend half the time for each compression pushing down and half the time letting the chest rise. Keep the compression cycles regular, smooth, and uninterrupted.

f. **Give Two Quick Breaths (3-5 seconds).** Immediately after giving the fifteenth chest compression, release the pressure, move your hands to the casualty's head, and open his airway. Close the nose (or mouth) and seal the casualty's mouth (or nose or stoma). Blow air in until the chest rises. Look out of the corner of your eye to be sure the chest rises. Break the seal, take a breath, and administer a second breath.

g. **Administer Three More Cardiopulmonary Resuscitation Cycles (15 Chest Compressions and Two Breaths Per Cycle).** Before you do this, relocate the compression site over the casualty's sternum. Use the procedure given in paragraph 2-13 i (l). <u>DO NOT</u> GUESS where the site is.

h. **Check the Pulse (3-5 seconds).**

(1) <u>Check the pulse after the first 4 CPR cycles</u>. If the pulse is absent, give two breaths and resume one-rescuer CPR. If the pulse is present, perform rescue breathing.

(2) Recheck the pulse every few (3-5) minutes after the initial pulse check.

Section IV. ONE-RESCUER METHOD CARDIOPULMONARY RESUSCITATION

1-13. INTRODUCTION

There are two basic methods of administering CPR. The one-rescuer method is used when you have no one available to help you perform CPR. The two-rescuer method is used when you have assistance available. The one-rescuer method is presented in this section, and the two-rescuer method is presented in Section V.

1-14. **ONE-RESCUER CARDIOPULMONARY RESUSCITATION METHOD**

This method should be taught to a lay person. Teaching two-rescuer CPR to a nonprofessional may only confuse him. One person alone can maintain sufficient circulation and ventilation, but doing this procedure alone is very tiring.

a. **Airway.**

(1) Determine that the casualty is unresponsive. Tap him on the shoulder, the shoulder nearest you. Gently shake him, taking care not to cause more injury. Shout, "Are you O.K.?" If the casualty does not respond, consider that he is unconscious. See figure 1-11.

(2) Call for help.

(3) Position the casualty, if necessary. Place the casualty on his back and on a flat, firm surface. Turn the casualty's body as a unit being careful not to injure his head or neck as you move him. When the casualty is on his back, put his arms by the side of his body.

(4) Kneel at the casualty's shoulders so that rescue breathing and chest compressions can be performed without the rescuer moving his own knees.

(5) Open the airway using the head-lilt/chin-lift method (figure 1-12).

b. **Breathing.** Begin assessment by determining whether the casualty is breathing.

(1) If the casualty is breathing, follow this procedure:

(a) Monitor the casualty's breathing.

(b) Keep the casualty's airway open.

(c) Yell for help.

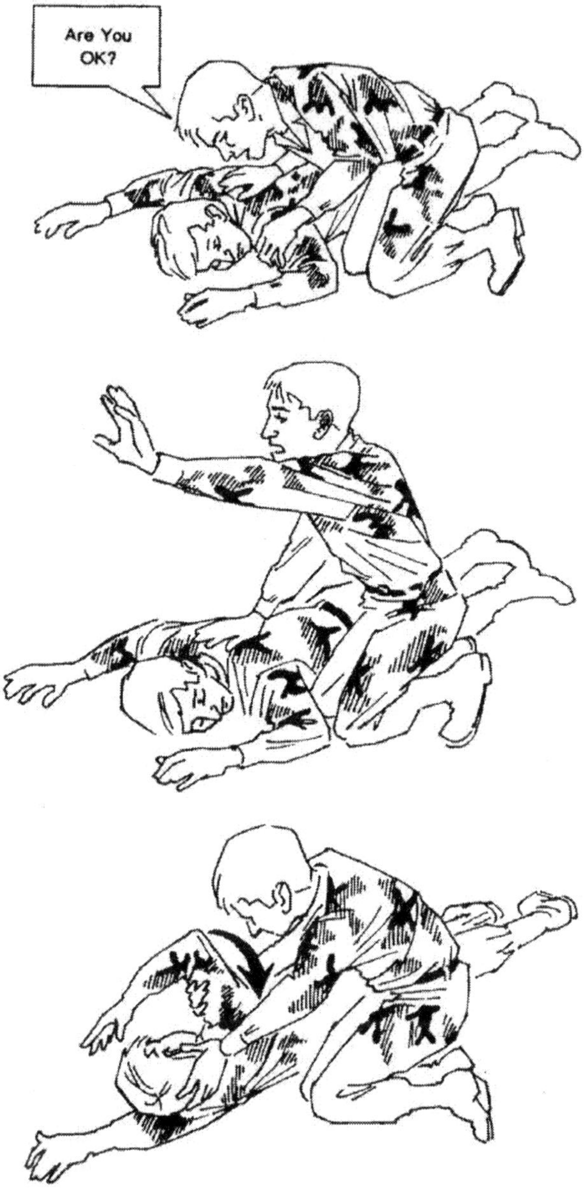

Figure 1-11. Initial steps of one-rescuer CPR.

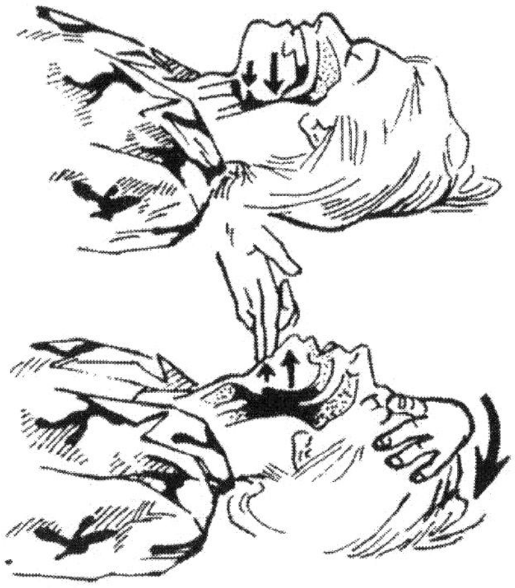

Figure 1-12. Head-tilt/chin-lift method.

(2) If the casualty is NOT breathing, follow this procedure:

(a) Begin rescue breathing by giving two full breaths.

(b) If you cannot give two full breaths, reposition the casualty's head. Try giving two full breaths again.

(c) If the attempt at ventilation is still unsuccessful, assume there is a foreign body in the airway. Clear the airway as you would if there were a foreign body in the airway. Then, ventilate with two full breaths. If this is successful, continue to the next step.

c. **Circulation.** Begin with assessment and determine whether the casualty has a pulse.

(1) Continue rescue breathing at the rate of 12 times per minute if there is a pulse.

(2) If there is no pulse, start external chest compressions using this procedure:

(a) Determine the correct hand position.

(b) Do 15 external chest compressions. The rate should be 80 to 100 chest compressions per minute. To get the proper rhythm and be sure you are performing the correct number of chest compressions, count one-and, two-and, three-and, four-and, five-and, six-and, seven-and, eight-and, nine-and, ten-and, eleven-and, twelve-and, thirteen-and, fourteen-and, fifteen."

(c) Open the casualty's airway. Give him two rescue breaths (full, slow breaths).

(d) Determine the proper hand position. Start 15 more external chest compressions at a rate of 80 to 100 chest compressions per minute.

(e) Do four complete cycles of 15 compressions and two ventilations.

d. **Reassessment.** Reassess the casualty after four cycles of compressions and ventilations.

(1) Check to see if the casualty's carotid pulse has returned. (It should take about 5 seconds to check.) If the casualty still has no pulse, begin CPR again by giving two ventilations then 15 compressions. If the casualty's pulse has resumed, go to the next step.

(2) Check to see if the casualty is breathing. (This check should take from 3 to 5 seconds.) If the casualty is breathing, check his breathing and pulse closely. If the casualty is NOT breathing, start rescue breathing at 12 times per minute. Also, monitor the pulse closely.

(3) If it is necessary to continue CPR, stop and check every few minutes to see if the casualty's pulse has started and if he has begun breathing again. Be careful not to stop CPR for more than 7 seconds at a time unless something very unusual is happening.

NOTE: One-rescuer CPR is summarized in figure 1-13.

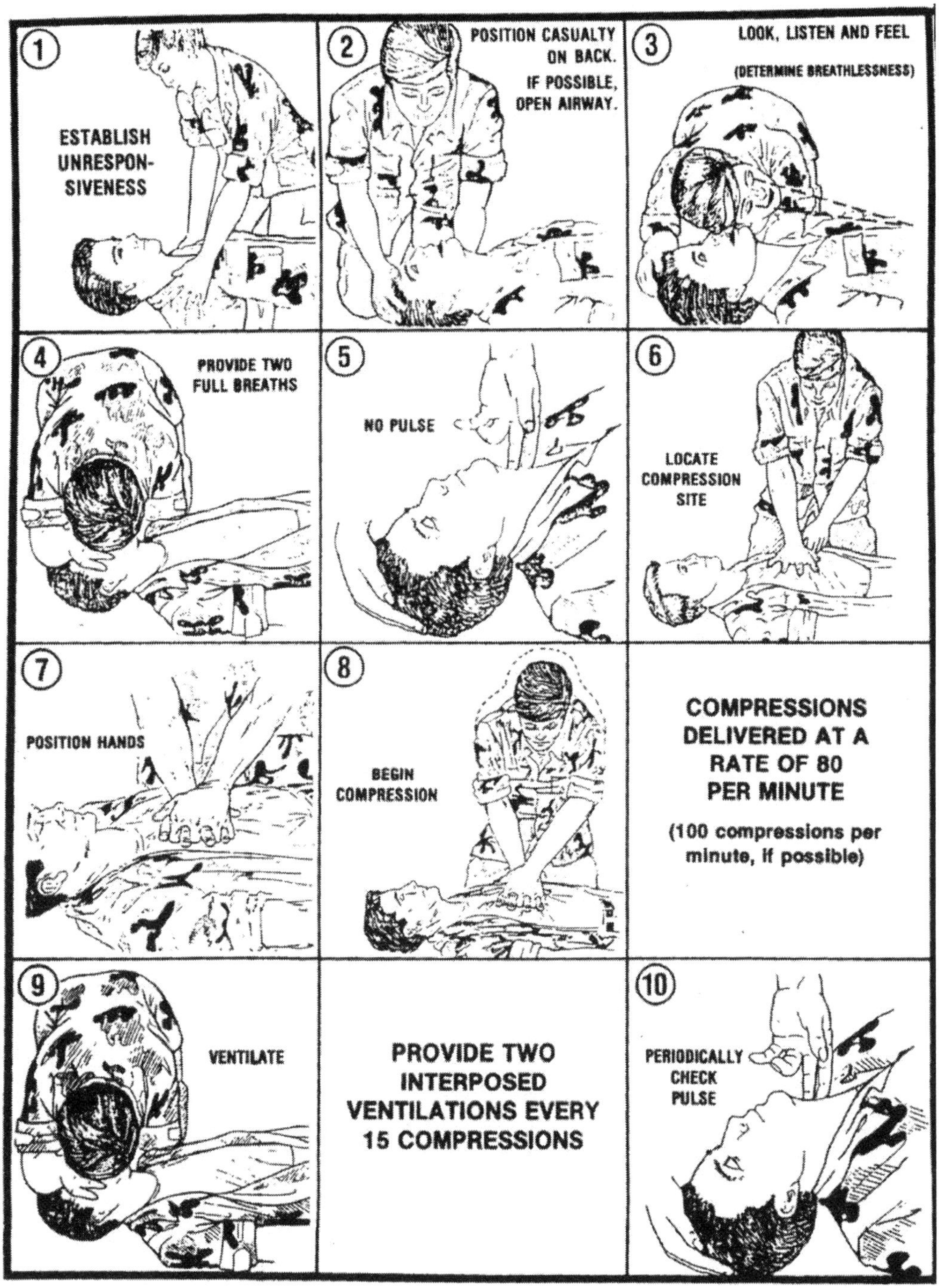

Figure 1-13. One-rescuer CPR.

Section V. TWO-RESCUER METHOD CARDIOPULMONARY RESUSCITATION

1-15. INTRODUCTION

If two rescuers are available, one rescuer can perform chest compressions while the other rescuer performs rescue breathing. One rescuer should position himself on one side of the casualty near his head while the other rescuer positions himself on the other side of the casualty near the casualty's chest.

1-16. TWO-RESCUER CARDIOPULMONARY RESUSCITATION: GENERAL METHOD

These general procedures are followed:

a. One rescuer positions himself at the casualty's side. He performs external chest compressions and may be called the <u>compressor</u>.

b. The other rescuer positions himself at the casualty's head. He may be called the <u>ventilator</u>. His responsibilities include:

(1) Maintaining an open airway.

(2) Monitoring the carotid pulse.

(3) Performing rescue breathing.

c. The compression rate for two-person CPR is 80 to 100 chest compressions per minute.

d. Five external chest compressions are given by one rescuer (the compressor), then two full breaths are given by the other rescuer (the ventilator). After the fifth compression, the compressor should pause 1 to 1 1/2 seconds for the ventilator to give the two full breaths. Five external chest compressions to one ventilation (two full breaths) is the ratio.

e. The two rescuers should change places when the compressor becomes tired.

NOTE: Two-rescuer CPR is summarized in figure 1-14.

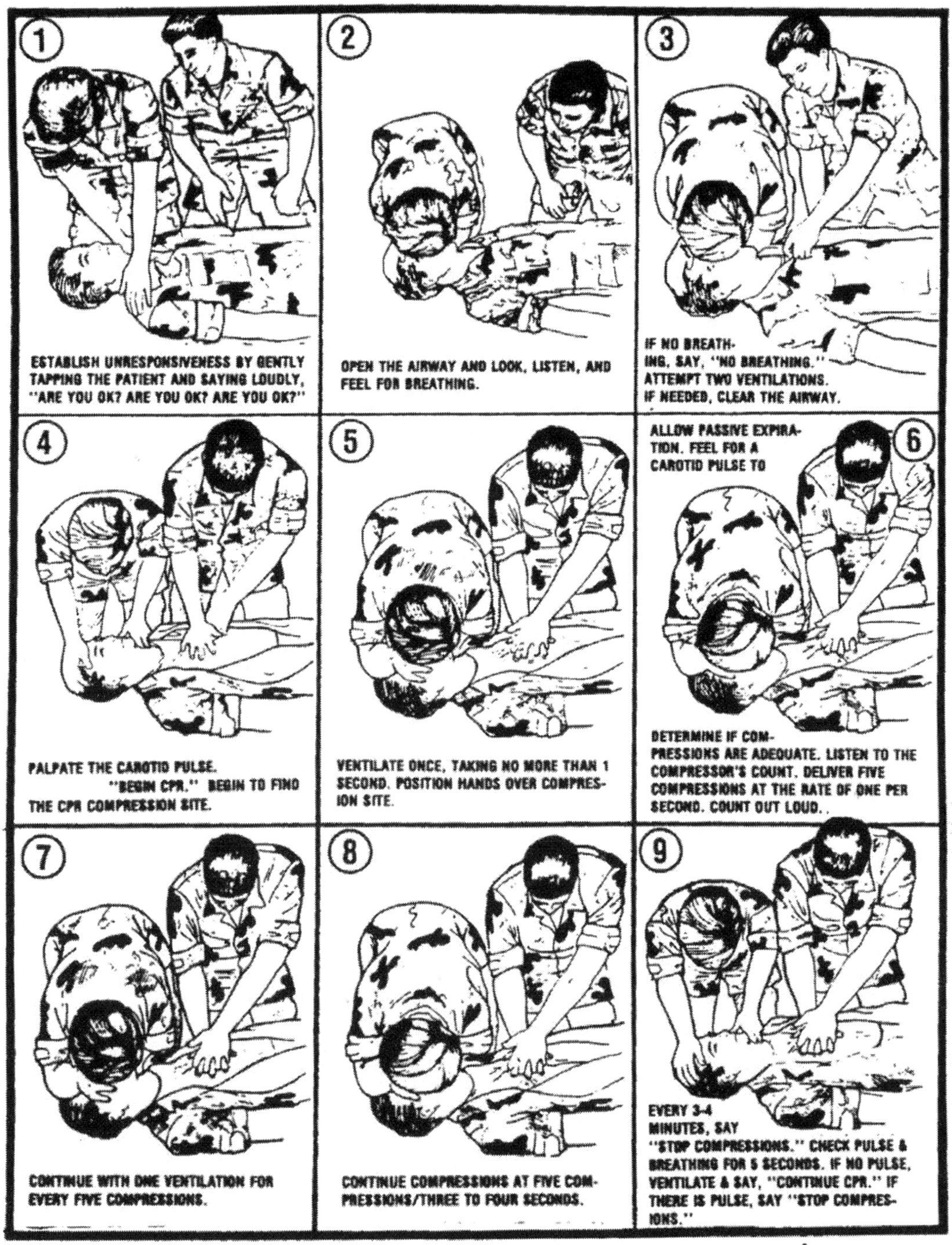

Figure 1-14. Two-rescuer CPR.

1-17. TWO-RESCUER CARDIOPULMONARY RESUSCITATION: ONE-RESCUER CARDIOPULMONARY RESUSCITATION IN PROGRESS

Cardiopulmonary resuscitation is being performed by one lay person, and two professional rescuers arrive at the same time. The rescuers enter the process just after the one rescuer has completed a cycle of 15 compressions and two breaths. (REMEMBER: One person doing CPR will perform fifteen external chest compressions then two full breaths. Two persons doing CPR will perform five external chest compressions then two full breaths.) Two rescuers follow this sequence of steps:

a. One rescuer (the ventilator) positions himself at the casualty's head. That rescuer (1) opens the airway and (2) checks for a pulse.

b. At the same time, the other rescuer (the compressor) positions himself at the casualty's side. This rescuer (1) locates the site for external chest compressions and (2) finds the proper hand position. Both the ventilator and the compressor's actions should take about 5 seconds.

c. If the ventilator finds no pulse, the compressor should begin external chest compressions at the rate of 80 to 100 per minute. The ventilator counts "one-and, two-and, three-and, four-and, five."

d. The compressor pauses at the end of five. The ventilator gives two full breaths.

NOTE: The pause for two full breaths may be shorter if a tube has been inserted to open the casualty's airway.

1-18. TWO-RESCUER CARDIOPULMONARY RESUSCITATION: NO CARDIOPULMONARY RESUSCITATION IN PROGRESS

When both rescuers arrive at the same time and no CPR is in progress, some decisions must be made. Both rescuers must decide what to do and start right away. They should follow this procedure:

a. Determine that the casualty is unresponsive.

b. Position the casualty.

c. One rescuer (the ventilator) should:

(1) Position himself at the casualty's head.

(2) Open the air-way.

(3) Check for breathing.

(4) If the casualty still is not breathing, say "No breathing" and give two full breaths.

(5) Check for carotid pulse. If there is no pulse, say "No pulse."

d. At the same time, the second rescuer (the compressor) should position himself by the casualty's side and:

(1) Find the site for external chest compressions.

(2) Place his hands in the correct position for external chest compressions.

(3) After the first rescuer says "No pulse", the compressor should begin external chest compressions.

e. The rescuers continue to administer CPR cycles (5 compressions and 2 breaths per cycle).

1-19. RESCUERS CHANGE POSITIONS IN TWO-RESCUER CARDIOPULMONARY RESUSCITATION

a. A position exchange (figure 1-15) is used to give tie rescuer at the chest a rest. If there are other CPR qualified persons in the area, a switch can be used to bring a new person in and take a tired rescuer out.

b. Follow this procedure to make a switch in rescuers:

(1) The first rescuer (person at the chest) initiates the exchange by counting, "Change-one thousand, two-one thousand, three-one thousand, four-one thousand, five-one thousand."

(2) Then, the second rescuer gives a breath and moves to the position for chest compressions while the first rescuer moves to the position for rescue breathing. The rescuers do not change sides.

(3) The first rescuer (now at the casualty's head) checks the casualty's pulse (takes about 5 seconds). If no pulse is felt, he tells the rescuer at the chest. The first rescuer continues to administer rescue breathing, and the second rescuer examines the casualty for injuries. If there is still no pulse during a second check, the rescuer at the chest is told. The other rescuer gives the casualty a breath, and both rescuers continue to administer CPR.

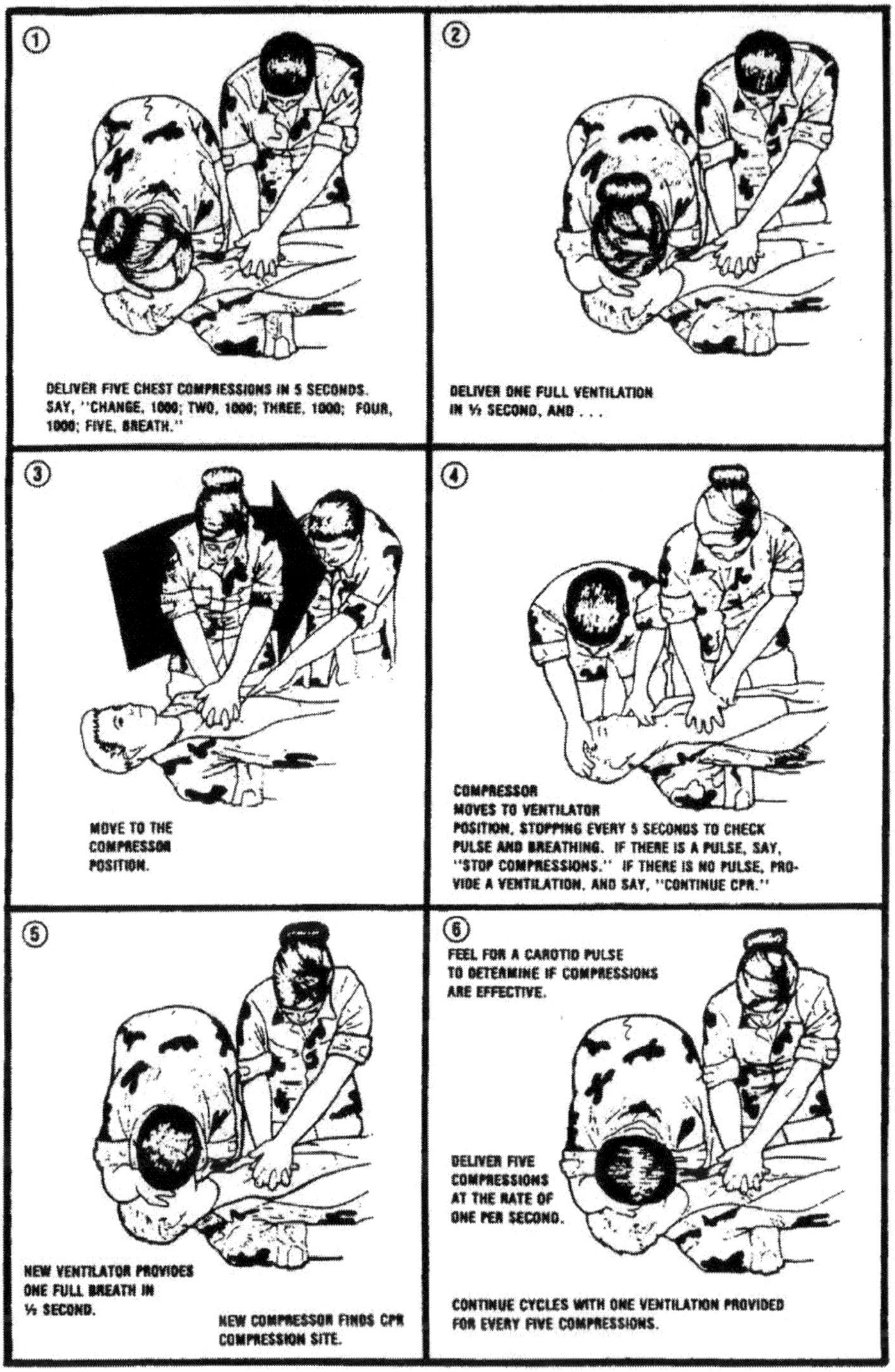

Figure 1-15. Rescuers change positions.

1-20. MONITOR THE CASUALTY

a. To be sure the CPR effort is effective, the casualty's condition must be monitored. The ventilator monitors the pulse and breathing to determine whether the chest compressions are effective and whether the casualty's circulation and breathing have begun gain.

b. The ventilator also checks the carotid pulse during chest compressions to determine if the chest compressions are effective.

c. At the end of the first minute and every few minutes after that, stop chest compressions for about 5 seconds to see if the casualty is breathing on his own and if his circulation has improved.

d. Rescuers should change places when the compressor is tired.

Section VI. CARDIOPULMONARY RESUSCITATION COMPLICATIONS/ CARDIOPULMONARY RESUSCITATION TERMINATION

1-21. CARDIOPULMONARY RESUSCITATION COMPLICATIONS

External chest compression and rescue breathing must be performed properly in order to support life. Sometimes even correctly performed CPR may cause complications.

a. **Neck and Spine Complications.** If the head is not positioned properly, you may not be able to get air into the casualty's lungs. You may, in fact, even cause neck and spine complications if the head is not in the proper position.

b. **Gastric Complications.** Too much air pushed too fast into the casualty can result in gastric distention (the air enters the casualty's stomach and pushes the stomach out). Gastric distention can be caused by the rescuer delivering the breaths with too much force, or the condition can be caused by an obstruction in the casualty's airway which prevents his lungs from filling quickly. Gastric distention can cause vomiting and may decrease the lung volume by pushing up on the diaphragm. The treatment for gastric distention is to recheck and reposition the casualty's head to be sure the airway is open. Ventilate and watch for the rise and fall of the casualty's chest. If ventilations are still inadequate, roll the casualty onto one side, press into his epigastrium (pit of the stomach), wipe out his mouth, and continue cardiopulmonary resuscitation.

CAUTION: Do not push on the casualty's abdomen.

c. **Fractures.** Fractures of the ribs or sternum may occur even if CPR is performed correctly. Care should be taking, however, to be sure there is proper hand placement and technique because fractures of the ribs or sternum (including the xyphoid process) can lead to punctured lungs; lacerated liver, aorta, stomach, or spleen; or cardiac tamponade (blood in the pericardial sac) caused by a lacerated pericardium.

d. **Vomiting (Regurgitation).** If the casualty vomits, turn his entire body onto one side and wipe out his mouth. Then, return him to the supine (flat on his back) position and continue administering CPR.

e. **Dentures.** Do not remove dentures from the casualty's mouth unless they are loose or broken. If it is necessary to remove dentures, send them with the casualty when he is evacuated (put them in his pocket, and so forth).

1-22. CARDIOPULMONARY RESUSCITATION TERMINATION

Generally, these are the only reasons to stop CPR: the rescuer is physically unable to continue, the rescuer is relieved by a doctor or other medical personnel, a doctor pronounces the casualty dead, or the casualty revives.

Continue with Exercises

EXERCISES, LESSON 1

INSTRUCTIONS: The following exercises are to be answered by writing the answer in the space provided. After you have completed all the exercises, turn to "Solutions to Exercises" at the end of the lesson and check your answers.

1. Sudden death may be defined as ______________________________

   ____

2. List two characteristics of clinical death.

   a. ______________________________________.

   b. ______________________________________.

3. What is biological death? ______________________________

   ____.

4. List three common causes of sudden death.

   a. ______________________________________.

   b. ______________________________________.

   c. ______________________________________.

5. List the two basic responsibilities of a rescuer during cardiopulmonary resuscitation.

   a. ______________________________________.

   b. ______________________________________.

6. Cardiopulmonary resuscitation means restoring ____________function and

   ____________________ function to a person who is clinical dead.

7. A person who is not breathing will die in a short time because ______________

____.

8. Cardiopulmonary resuscitation is made up of rescue breathing

and ____

9. The head-tilt/chin-lift method and the jaw thrust methods are both methods of

____ during rescue breathing.

10. When you are checking for breathing during rescue breathing, you should look at the casualty's is chest to see if ________________________________, listen for _________________________, and feel for __________________________.

11. Mouth-to-stoma rescue breathing is used when the casualty ________________

____.

12. Rescue breathing is part of CPR in which an unconscious casualty is forced to

____.

13. List four reasons cardiopulmonary resuscitation may be stopped.

a. ____.

b. ____.

c. ____.

d. ____.

14. When you are giving chest compressions, a compression cycle consists of

_________________________________ which compresses the heart and

___________________________ which allows the heart to refill with blood.

15. When two people have knowledge of CPR, one rescuer can perform

_____________________________ and the other rescuer can perform the

____.

16. When checking for the casualty's pulse during CPR, check the carotid pulse

because _________________________ and you are already near the neck.

17. You cannot feel the casualty's pulse and you are preparing to administer chest

compressions. The first thing you do is _______________________________.

Check Your Answers on Next Page

SOLUTIONS TO EXERCISES, LESSON 1

1. The unexpected cessation of respiration and functional circulation. (para 1-2)

2. Heartbeat has stopped.
   Breathing has stopped. (para 1-2a)

3. Biological death is permanent cellular damage due to lack of oxygen. (para 1-2b)

4. You are correct if you listed any three of the following:

   Drowning
   Choking on food or other objects
   Electrical shock
   Poisoning
   Sensitivity reaction and anaphylactic shock
   Suffocation
   Smoke inhalation.
   Automobile accident.
   Myocardial infarction
   Medical reasons. (para 1-4a through j)

5. Prevent biological death.
   Get competent help. (para 1-5)

6. Lung.
   Heart. (para 1-6)

7. The cells are not receiving a fresh supply of oxygen. (para 1-8)

8. Chest compressions. (para 1-10)

9. Establishing an airway. (paras 1-9c(l) and (2))

10. The chest rises and falls.
    The sound of breathing.
    The flow of air on the side of your face. (paras 1-9d(l) through (4))

11. Has had his larynx surgically removed leaving an opening in the neck for breathing. (para 1-9f, NOTE)

12. Inhale and exhale. (para 1-9f)

13. The rescuer is physically exhausted and can't continue.
    The rescuer is relieved by a doctor or another rescuer.
    The doctor pronounces the casualty dead.
    The casualty revives. (para 1-22)

14. A thrust.
    A release. (para 1-12c(4))

15. Chest compressions.
    Rescue breathing. (para 1-15)

16. A carotid pulse can sometimes be felt when other pulses are too weak to be detected. (para 1-9f(1)(d))

17. Locate the compression site. (para 1-12a)

End of Lesson 1

LESSON ASSIGNMENT

LESSON 2 Dysrhythmia Recognition and Treatment.

LESSON ASSIGNMENT Paragraphs 2-1 through 2-12.

LESSON OBJECTIVES After completing this lesson, you should be able to:

2-1. Identify electrocardiogram rhythms.

2-2. Identify normal sinus rhythm.

2-3. Identify and treat these cardiac dysrhythmias:

Sinus bradycardia.
Sinus tachycardia.
Wandering pacemaker.
Premature atrial contractions.
Atrial tachycardia.
Atrial flutter.
Atrial fibrillation.
Premature junctional contraction.
First-degree heart block.
Wenckebach heart block.
Classical second-degree heart block.
Complete heart block.
Premature ventricular contractions.
Ventricular tachycardia.
Ventricular fibrillation.
Idioventricular rhythm.
Asystole.

SUGGESTION After completing the assignment, complete the exercises of this lesson. These exercises will help you to achieve the lesson objectives.

LESSON 2

DYSRHYTHMIA RECOGNITION AND TREATMENT

Section I. DYSRHYTHMIA

2-1. INTRODUCTION

a. Dysrhythmia is a disturbance in cardiac rhythm. Ninety percent of patients with acute myocardial infarction (heart attack) will experience a form of cardiac dysrhythmia during the first couple of weeks after their attack. Half of these will be life threatening and will lead to cardiac arrest (sudden stoppage of adequate cardiac output) unless properly treated. In order to analyze and treat a dysrhythmia correctly, you must have a systematic approach to the electrocardiogram (EKG). Only after this process has been completed can you make sound judgments as to which cardiac drug to administer and when to defibrillate or use cardioversion.

b. When monitoring a patient's EKG, remember that you are monitoring electrical activity of a heart, not mechanical activity. So, a pulse is always taken to assure you of the heart's pumping action. Information learned from the EKG will be used to help determine the treatment of the dysrhythmia. Dysrhythmia treatment could be defibrillation, cardioversion, intravenous cardiac drugs, and/or CPR.

DYSRHYTHMIA = a disturbance in cardiac rhythm.
ELECTROCARDIOGRAM = monitors electrical activity of the heart.

2-2. DYSRHYTHMIA CAUSES/SIGNIFICANCE

a. **Causes of Dysrhythmia.** Dysrhythmias develop for various reasons including acute myocardial infarction (heart attack), trauma, and drug reactions. Drowning, near drowning, asphyxiation, and the patient's underlying medical conditions can also cause dysrhythmias.

b. **Significance of Dysrhythmia.** There are several reasons why cardiac dysrhythmias may be clinically significant. Heart rates below 40 to 50 beats per minute lead to inadequate cardiac output and often precede electric instability of the heart. If the sinus rate falls below 60 beats per minute, another conduction system may take over. The Atrial Ventricular Junction (AV Junction) has an inherent rate of 40 to 60 beats a minute. The Ventricle has an inherent rate of 20 to 40 beats a minute. This may lead to premature ventricular contractions and ventricular dysrhythmias. If a heart rate is over 120 to 140 beats per minute, the heart must work harder. This causes further myocardial ischemia (diminished blood flow). Tachycardias may be linked with a drop in cardiac output which is secondary to decreased stroke volume, this lowered volume being caused by the ventricles having less time to fill between heartbeats. And, finally, ectopic beats (beats located away from the normal position) could be a sign of electric instability of the ventricles. Such heartbeats are an important sign since they may indicate that more serious dysrhythmias such as ventricular tachycardia or ventricular fibrillation may develop.

Section II. ELECTROPHYSIOLOGY

2-3. GENERAL

a. **Heart Cells.** Two types of cells are found in the heart: electrical cells and mechanical cells. The heart's conduction system is mare-up of electrical cells. These cells have the ability to begin and transmit electrical activity in the heart. Myocardial cells (the mechanical cells) make up the bulk musculature of the heart. When an electrical stimuli reaches these cells, the cells contract. An electrical impulse stimulates the mechanical action of the heart causing the heart to pump effectively. If the electrical system of the heart does not function properly, arrhythmias (a mechanical activity) may occur.

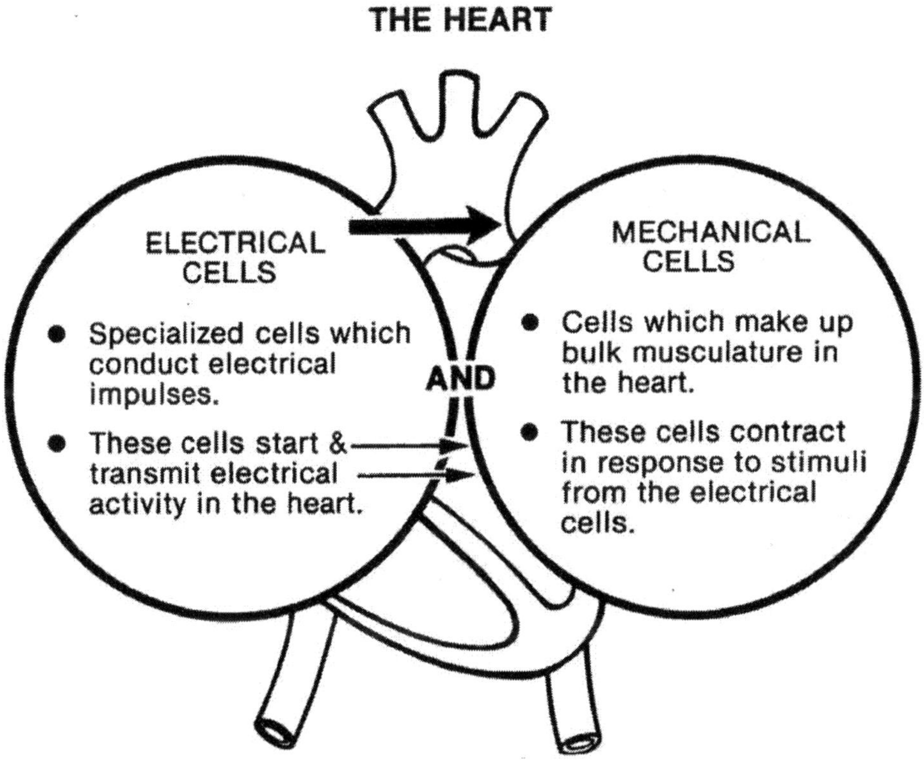

Figure 2-1. Electrical cells and mechanical cells.

b. **Electrical Activity In The Heart.** The heart's electrical activity begins in the sinoatrial (SA) node and flows toward the ventricles. See figure 3-2. All the areas of this conduction system can do the following: initiate impulses; become irritable; respond to an impulse. Impulses are initiated in each area of the conduction system as shown here:

SA node ....60-100 per minute
AV Junction......40-60 per minute
Ventricle ....20-40 per minute

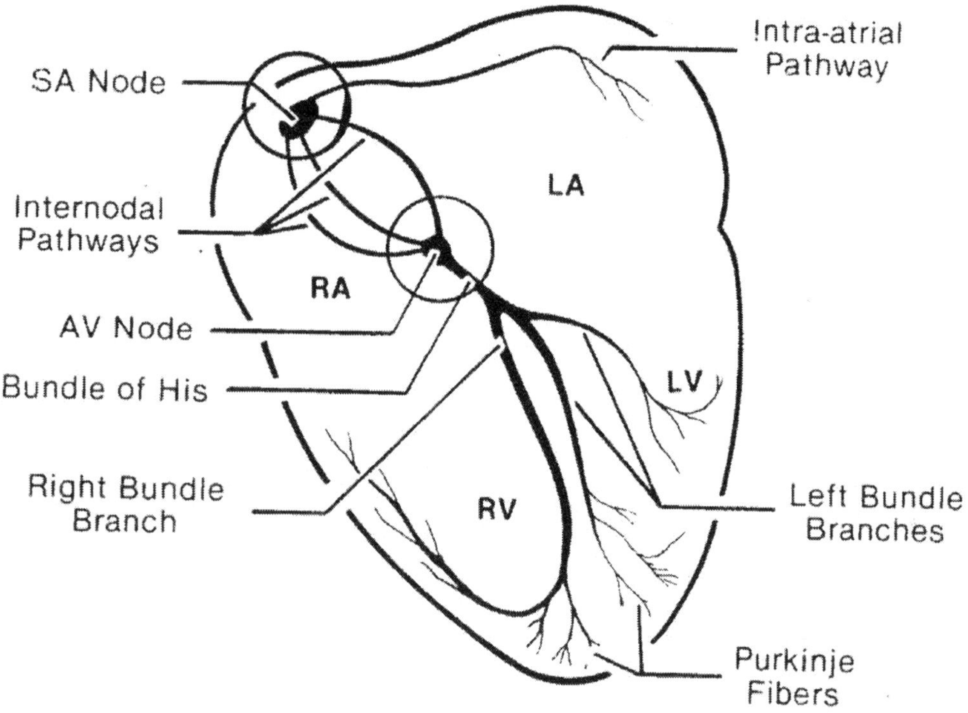

Figure 2-2. Electrical conduction system of the heart.

c. **The Pacemaker Site.** The common pacemaker site is the SA node because it initiates electrical impulses at a faster rate than the junction or ventricle. An impulse from the AV junction can take over if the SA node should fail. If the AV junction also fails, the ventricle can take over. This is a protective backup system, a system which helps the heart maintain electrical efficiency. Sometimes the junction or the ventricle becomes irritable and starts impulses at a faster than normal rate which overrides the SA node. When this happens, the pacemaker site that is the fastest dominates and takes over control of the heart.

2-4. INNERVATION

The autonomic nervous system (ANS) regulates internal organ activities, usually involuntarily and automatically. This system regulates sweating, alters the size of the pupils, and directs many other body adjustments. The ANS influences the heart rate and myocardial contractility (the ability of cardiac muscle cells or tissues to shorten when stimulated) by sympathetic and/or parasympathetic stimulation. Sympathetic impulses increase heart activity; parasympathetic impulses decrease heart activity. Both of these systems must be in balance for the heart to function properly. If one or the other system is stimulated abnormally or blocked, the result will be heart arrhythmias. See figure 2-3 for autonomic nervous system control of the heart.

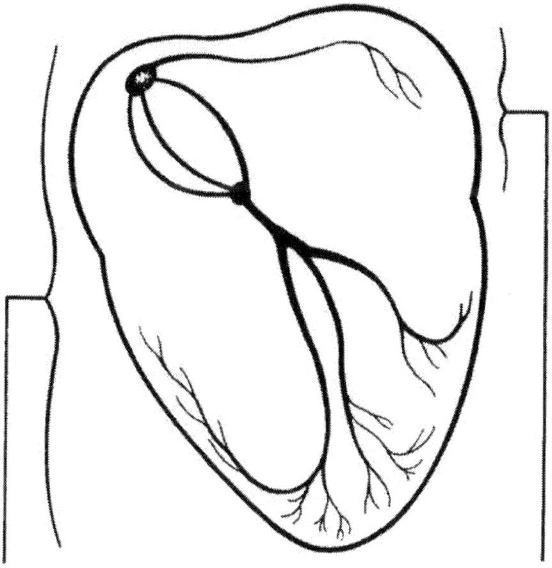

SYMPATHETIC

- Innervates both atria and ventricles
- Increases
  Heart Rate
  AV Conduction
  Irritability

PARASYMPATHETIC

- Innervates the atria via vagus nerve
- Little or no effect on junction or ventricles
- Decreases
  Heart Rate
  AV Conduction
  Irritability

Figure 2-3. Innervation of the heart.

2-5. **GRAPHIC DISPLAY OF ELECTROCARDIOGRAM**

a. **Heart Electrical Forces.** During the cardiac cycle (one contraction of the heart plus the relaxation period that follows), electrical changes take place in the heart. These changes can be visualized and recorded.

(1) Detection of electrical forces in the heart. Electrical forces in the heart can be detected on the body's surface. Therefore, electrodes attached to the patient's skin can detect electrical forces in the heart.

(2) Recording of electrical forces in the heart. The recording of the electrical changes during the cardiac cycle is called an electrocardiogram (ECG or EKG). The instrument used to record these changes is an electrocardiograph.

b. **Electrocardiogram Graph Paper and Machines.** Electrocardiogram graph paper and the speed of the EKG machines are standard and uniform. Lines on the graph paper are horizontal and vertical with four light lines between two heavy lines. The horizontal lines indicate voltage. The electrical voltage of the heart impulse is measured in millivolts and determined by the magnitude of deflection (the power of a wave).

(1) Determination of electrical impulse strength. Compare the height of a wave spike to the horizontal lines to determine the strength of the electrical impulse.

(2) Vertical lines. Vertical lines indicate the speed of the electrical current traveling within the heart. The distance in time between two heavy vertical lines is 0.20 seconds and between two light vertical lines or across one small square is 0.04 seconds.

(3) Heavy lines. Heavy lines are necessary to determine rates, rules, and normal values. Light lines are composed of five small columns between two heavy vertical lines.

(4) Squares. There are 25 squares in each large square.

(5) Standard rate of EKG paper. The standard rate of EKG paper travels past the stylus at a rate of millimeters per second.

(6) Graph paper markings. The markings on the graph paper can be examined and compared to normal markings to give the reader an idea of the electrical activity of the patient's heart. See figure 2-4 for an example of standard EKG graph paper measurements.

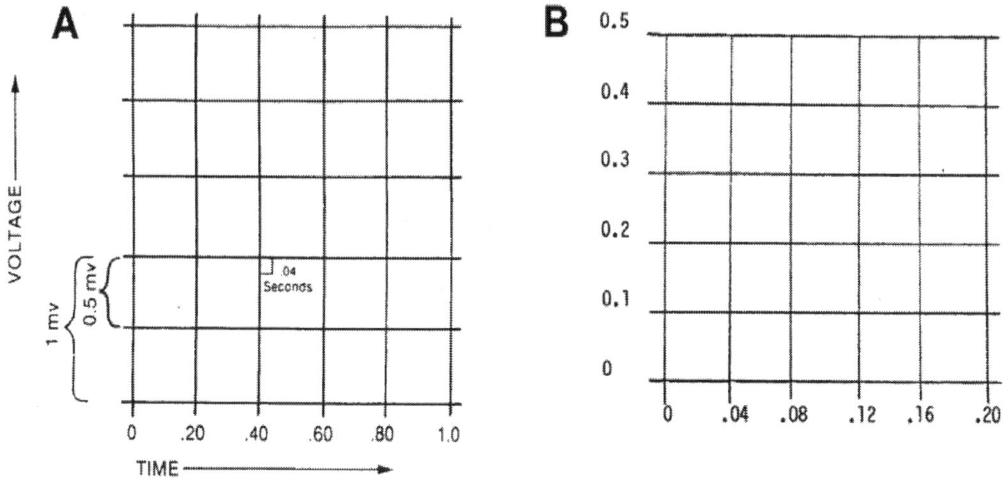

Figure 2-4. Standard graph paper measurements. A Graph paper. B Enlargemen of one square of graph paper.

c. **Electrical Impulses of Electrocardiogram Waves.** Each part of the cardiac cycle produces a different electrical impulse. The electrical flow of the heart starts with the SA node (right atrium) and continues to the Purkinje fibers (ventricles). Electrodes transmit impulses to a recording pen which graphs the impulses in a series of up and down waves called deflection waves. The cardiac cycle includes all of the wave patterns produced by electrical activity beginning with the pacemaker impulses and including ventricular repolarization. An isoelectric line occurs when there is no current strong enough to produce either a positive or negative deflection. The positive and negative forces are equal with the result that a flat line is shown (usually following the "T" wave). An electrical force (from the heart) toward the positive electrode will draw the stylus in an upright wave while an electrical force toward the negative electrode will draw the stylus in a downward wave. A single cardiac cycle is expected to produce one heartbeat. Deflections above or below the isoelectric line are called waves. Each wave is labeled with a letter. The waves are called the P wave, QRS complex, and the T wave. The letters were arbitrarily selected and do not stand for any words. Here are the waves:

(1) P wave. A small upward (positive) wave that indicates atrial polarization (the spread of an impulse from the SA node through the muscle of the two atria). The atria contract a fraction of a second after the P wave begins.

(2) QRS wave (complex). This second wave begins as a downward deflection and continues as a large, upright, triangular wave which finally ends as a downward wave at its base. This wave complex shows the spread of the electrical impulse through the ventricles.

(3) T wave. The third wave showing ventricular repolarization.

NOTE: There is no deflection to show atrial repolarization because the stronger QRS wave masks this event.

NOTE: Figure 2-5 shows EKG wave patterns produced by the electrical activity of the heart.

Electrical Activity	Graphic Depiction	Associated Pattern
Atrial Depolarization	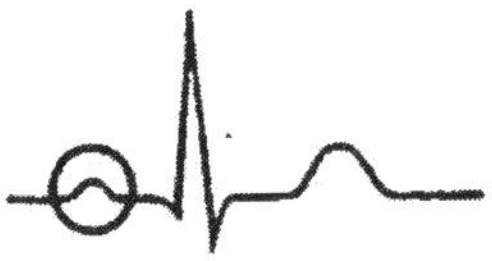	P Wave
Delay at AV Node	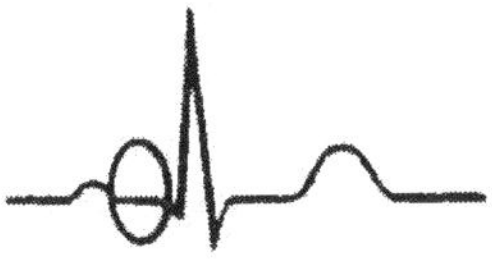	PR Segment
Ventricular Depolarization	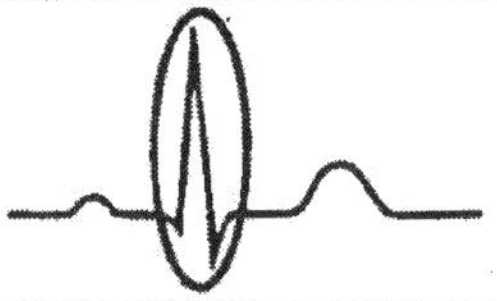	QRS Complex
Ventricular Repolarization	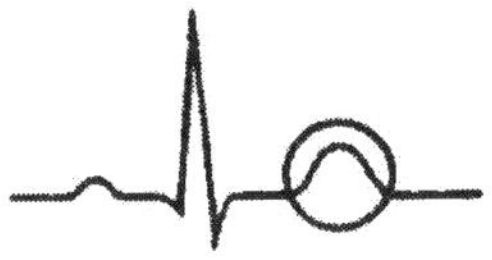	T Wave
No electrical activity	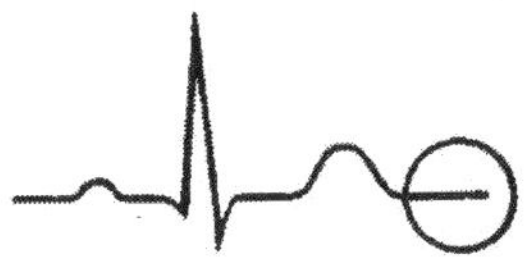	Isoelectric Line

Figure 2-5. Electrocardiogram wave patterns produced by electrical activity in the heart.

d. **Size and Time Intervals of EKG Waves.** The size of the deflection waves and particular time intervals are important when you are reading an electrocardiogram. For example, the duration of a normal "P" wave is between 0.06 and 0.1 seconds, the time it takes for depolarization current to pass through the atrial musculature. An increased width of "P" wave may indicate left atrial abnormality or right atrial hypertrophy (enlargement). The deflection of a normal "P" wave is small due to the thin walled structure of the atria. A "P" wave is usually no more than 3 mm high. A taller "P" wave may indicate that atrial enlargement has occurred due to hypertension, coronary pulmonade, or congenital heart disease.

(1) P-R interval. Measured from the beginning of the P wave to the beginning of the R wave, this wave pattern represents the conduction time from the beginning of atrial excitation to the beginning of ventricular excitation. This is the time it takes for an electrical impulse to travel through the atria and atrioventricular node to the remaining conducting tissues. A medical condition that disrupts this electrical impulse will display itself as a P-R interval that is longer than 0.2 seconds, due to the increased time it takes to travel the conducting tissues. The normal P-R interval is between 0.12 and 0.20 seconds.

(2) Q wave. The Q wave is defined as the first down (negative) deflection following the P wave but coming before the R wave.

(3) QRS complex. This complex is made up of three waves: the Q, the R, and the S waves. The QRS complex represents ventricular depolarization. A normal QRS measurement is less than 0.12 seconds. The QRS complex is larger than the P wave on an EKG because ventricular depolarization involves a greater muscle mass than atrial depolarization.

(4) R wave. The R wave is the first upward (positive) deflection that follows the wave.

(5) S-T segment. Beginning at the end of the S wave ending at the beginning of the T wave, this wave represents the time between the end of the spread of the heart's electrical impulse through the ventricles and repolarization of the ventricles. When a patient has acute myocardial infarction, the S-T segment is elevated. When the heart muscle does not receive enough oxygen, the S-T segment is depressed.

(6) T wave. Representing repolarization of the ventricular cells, the T wave is flat when the heart muscle does not receive enough oxygen; for example, in atherosclerotic heart disease. When the body's potassium level is increased, the T wave may be elevated. This wave occurs after the QRS complex.

NOTE: Refer to figure 2-6 to see these waves.

EKG Component	Graphic Depiction	Definition
PR Segment	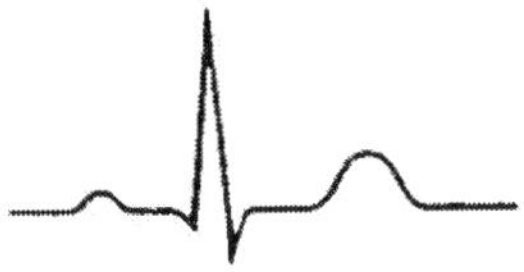	From the end of the P wave to the beginning of the QRS complex
PRI	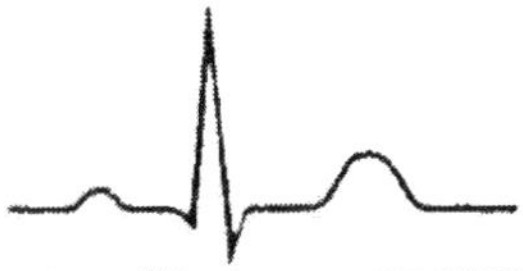	From the beginning of the P wave to the beginning of the QRS complex (normally .12 - .20 seconds)
Q Wave	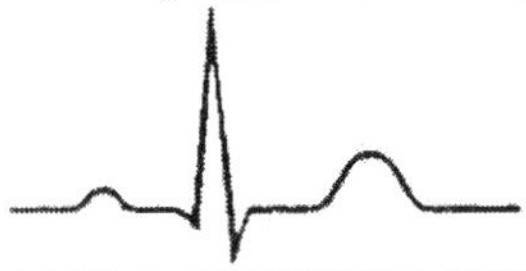	First negative deflection of the QRS complex
R Wave	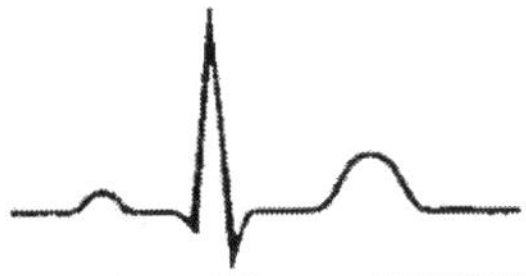	First positive deflection of the QRS complex
S Wave	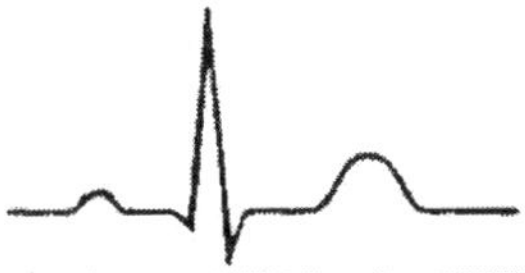	First negative deflection following the R wave
QRS Complex	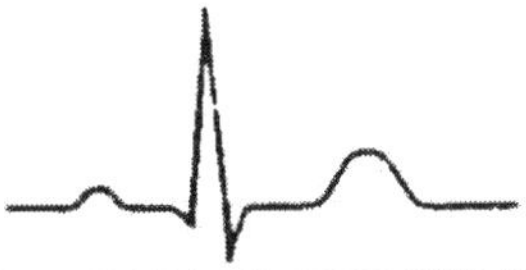	From the beginning of the Q wave to the end of the S wave (normally less than .12 seconds)
ST Segment	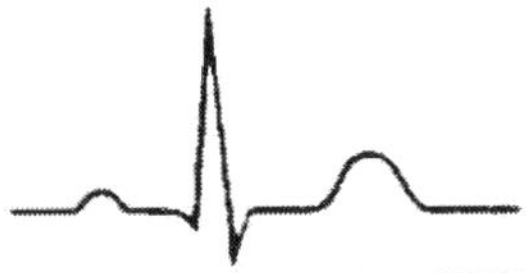	From the end of the S wave to the beginning of the T wave

Figure 2-6. EKG wave, segment, and internal definitions.

(7) The refractory period. During this period, cell charges are depolarized and have not returned to their polarized state. A cell that is electrically "refractory" cannot receive another impulse until it is repolarized. The refractory period on an EKG includes the QRS complex and the T wave. The absolute refractory period includes the QRS and the upslope of the T wave and is NOT a dangerous period. The relative refractory period may allow depolarization of ventricles. This period occurs on the downslope of the T wave; it is dangerous if an impulse occurs at this time.

e. **Electrocardiogram Uses.** The EKG has a variety of uses; for example, abnormal cardiac rhythms and conduction patterns and following the course of recovery from a heart attack. Some people carry a Holter monitor to monitor heart electrical activity. This machine can be carried around by the patient while he goes about his everyday routines. The Holter monitor is especially useful in detecting rhythm disorders in the conduction system. It is also useful in correlating rhythm disorders and symptoms and then following the effectiveness of drugs in dealing with these disorders.

Section III. RHYTHMS/HEART BLOCKS

2-6. ANALYSIS OF EKG RHYTHM STRIPS

a. **Regularity.**

(1) Determine regularity (also called rhythm) by looking at the R to R interval (RRI). This interval can be regular or irregular.

(2) The R-R interval is constant for regular rhythm, which means the distance between the beats, is the same.

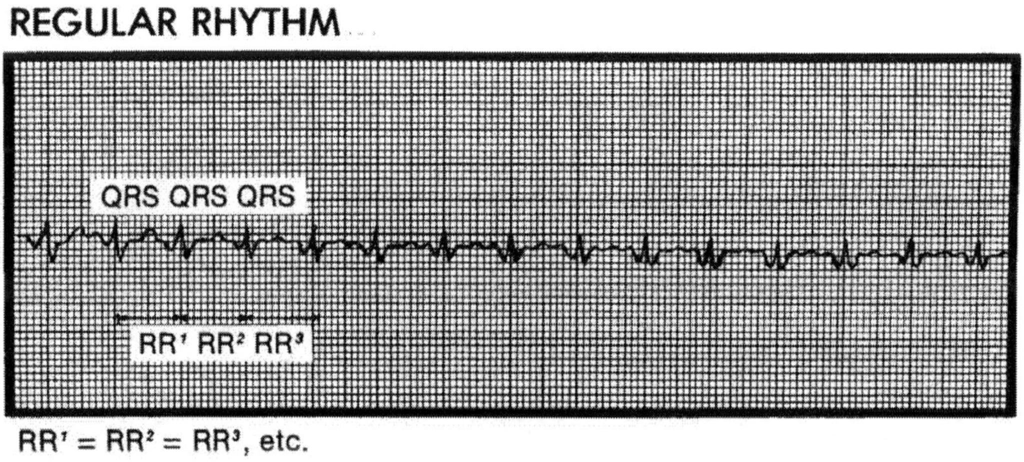

Figure 2-7. Regular rhythm.

(3) If the R to R interval (RRI) is inconsistent and the rhythm is irregular, the heartbeats are premature. A basically regular rhythm occurs when a heartbeat or two interrupt a regular rhythm; for example, ectopic (heartbeats originating from an abnormal place; that is, from somewhere other than the S-A node) or grouped heartbeats. A regularly irregular rhythm is a pattern of irregularity. A totally irregular rhythm has no pattern at all.

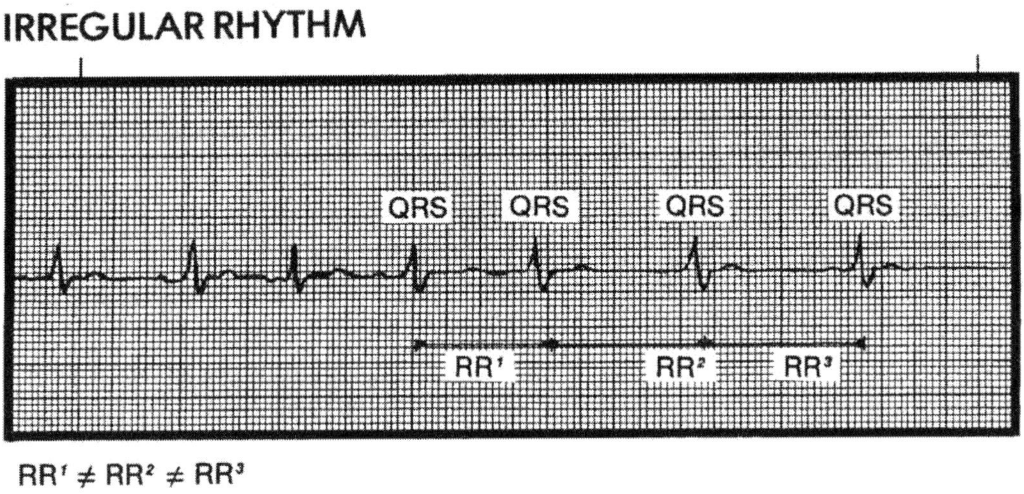

Figure 2-8. Irregular rhythm. (file: 5712-8.pcx)

b. **Rate.**

(1) Rate for regular heartbeat rhythms can be calculated in two ways.

(a) Method I. The most accurate method is to count the number of small squares between the two R waves and divide that number into 1500.

(b) Method II. The faster method is to count the number of large squares between R waves and divide that number into 300. This method is useful during an emergency. This method does not require a 6-second strip. Also, it allows rapid rate calculation using simple memorization of rate for large boxes. See figure 2-9.

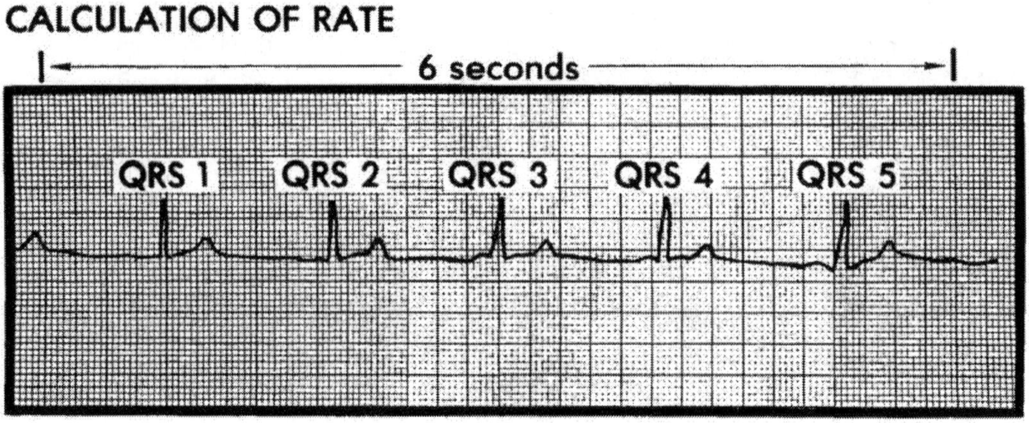

Figure 2-9. Calculation of heartbeat rate.

(2) The heartbeat rate for irregular heartbeat rhythm is based on the 6-second strip method. The minimum amount of time needed to determine cardiac rhythm is 6 seconds. The method described here is the quickest and easiest method although it is not as accurate as the "box" method. The vertical notches in the upper margin of the paper are 3 seconds apart.

(a) Count the number of QRS complexes in a 6-second strip.

(b) Multiply by 10 to get the heart rate for one minute.

c. **P Waves.** P waves are small positive deflections that occur on the oscilloscope. These waves represent atrial depolarization. Normally, the P waves are rounded, uniform, and upright and come before the QRS complex. These waves are either regular or irregular. Measured distances between all P waves should be constant. Determine whether there is a P wave for every QRS complex. Determine whether the P wave is in front of the QRS complex and see if there are more P waves than QRS complexes. Check to see if all the P waves look alike. See if there are irregular P waves associated with ectopic or irregular beats.

d. **P-R Intervals.** All P-R intervals should be constant. Measure the P-R intervals to determine if the intervals are normal or abnormal. A normal P-R interval is from 0.12 to 0.20 seconds. If the P-R interval varies, notice if there is a pattern to the changing measurements.

e. **QRS Complexes.** These complexes represent ventricular depolarization. The QRS complexes should be of equal duration.

(1) Here is an analysis of the parts of the QRS complex.

(a) Q waves are a negative deflection on the oscilloscope. They follow the P waves.

(b) R waves are a positive deflection on the oscilloscope, and they follow the Q waves.

(c) S waves are a negative deflection on the oscilloscope following the R waves.

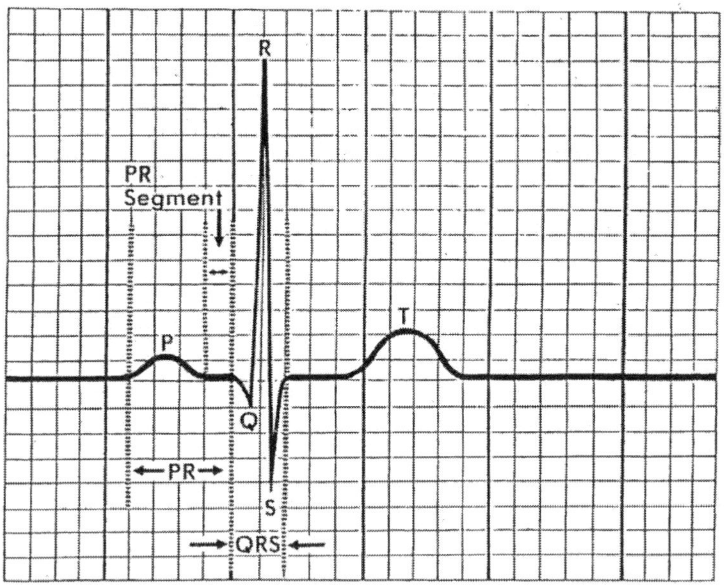

Figure 2-10. Electrocardiograph waves, segments, and intervals.

(2) Check the measurement of the QRS complex. The complex should be less than 0.12 seconds. See if the measurement is within normal limits. See if all the QRS complexes look alike. If there are any unusual QRS complexes, determine if they are associated with ectopic beats (abnormal heartbeats).

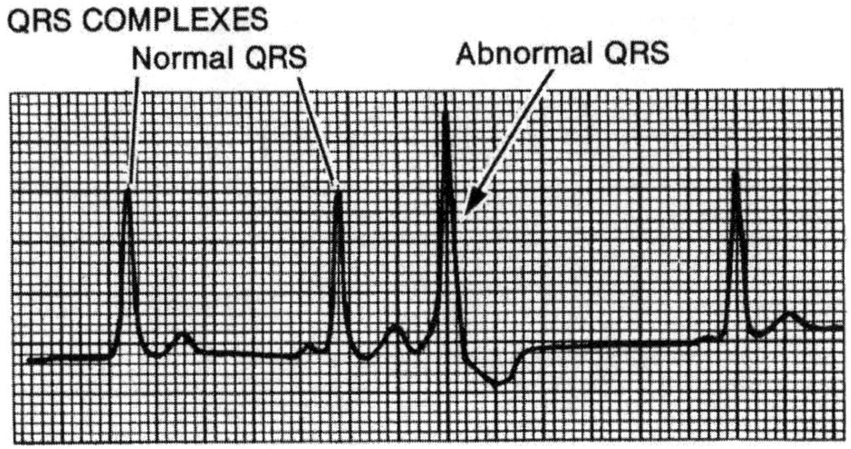

Figure 2-11. QRS complexes.

NOTE: For instructional purposes, the lines on the figures showing heartbeats are sometimes heavier than normal.

2-7. CARDIAC RHYTHMS

a. **Normal Sinus Rhythm (NSR).**

(1) Normal sinus rhythm originates in the SA node (pacemaker) and travels through the normal conduction pathways. It is not an arrhythmia (abnormality in the normal cardiac rhythm) or dysrhythmia (a disturbance in cardiac rhythm) because it is a normal pattern.

(2) Normal sinus rhythm is analyzed in this manner:

(a) When the R-R intervals and the P-P intervals are constant, the rhythm is considered regular.

(b) The atrial and ventricular rates equal 60 to 100 heartbeats per minute with no added or lost P, QRS, or T waves.

(c) The P wave has a uniform configuration with one P wave in front of every QRS.

(d) The P-R interval is constant between 0.12 and 0.20 seconds.

(e) The QRS complex measures less than 0.12 seconds.

(3) There is no treatment for normal sinus rhythm.

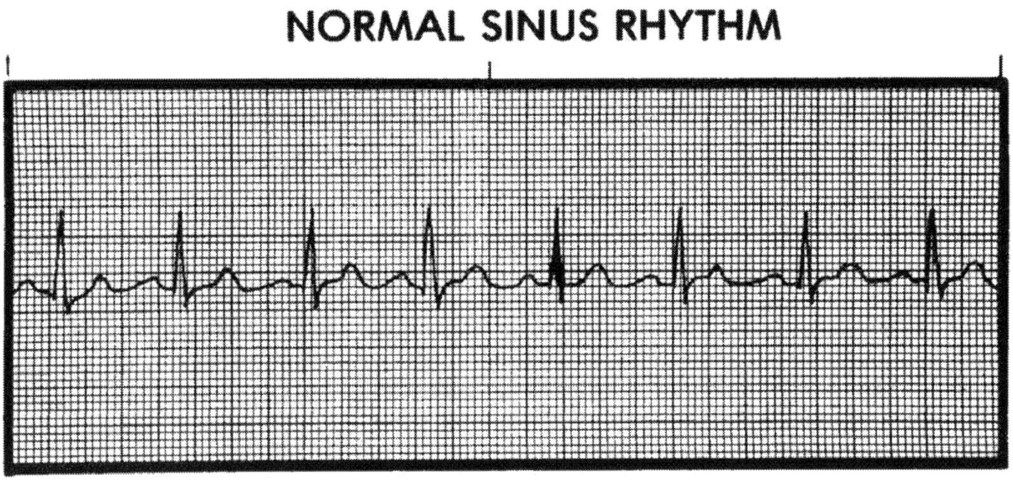

Figure 2-12. Normal sinus rhythm.

b. **Sinus Bradycardia.**

(1) Analysis.

(a) The rhythm is regular with the R-R intervals constant and the P-P intervals constant.

(b) The atrial and ventricular rates are less than 60 beats per minute.

(c) The P wave is normal and upright with one P wave in front of every QRS complex.

(d) The P-R interval is constant between 0.12 and 0.20 seconds.

(e) The QRS complex measures less than 0.12 seconds.

(f) A heart rate of less than 60 beats per minute may indicate good physical conditioning if the individual is young and healthy.

(g) If the person is suffering from acute myocardial infarction (AMI), this heartbeat rate may indicate any one of the following: conduction system damage, increased parasympathetic tone, or possible toxic levels of certain cardiac drugs (digitalis, quinidine). If the heartbeat rate decreases to less than 50 beats per minute, the heart may not be able to pump enough fluid through the body's vital organs. Additionally, bradycardia leads to electrical instability in the ventricles possibly resulting in ventricular arrhythmias.

NOTE: Males normally have a slower heart rate than females. Cardiovascularly healthy people may normally have a slow (less than 60 beats per minute) heart rate which also normally slows during sleep and rest. A slow heart rate is significant only if it is associated with MI or cardiovascular compromise.

(2) Treatment.

(a) There is no treatment if the casualty's blood pressure is normal, he is alert, and there are no ventricular, abnormal beats.

(b) If the casualty is experiencing premature ventricular contractions (PVCs), hypotension, or there are MI symptoms (chest pain or dyspnea), administer atropine. The dosage for a patient NOT in cardiac arrest is 0.5 mg intravenously at 5 minute intervals until the heart rate increases to 60 beats per minute or greater and until the signs and symptoms lessen. The dosage of atropine should not exceed 2 mg.

(c) Treat premature ventricular contractions (PVCs) with a bradycardiac rhythm) with atropine, NOT lidocaine. The reason is that atropine may restore the normal AV conduction system, but lidocaine may block this response.

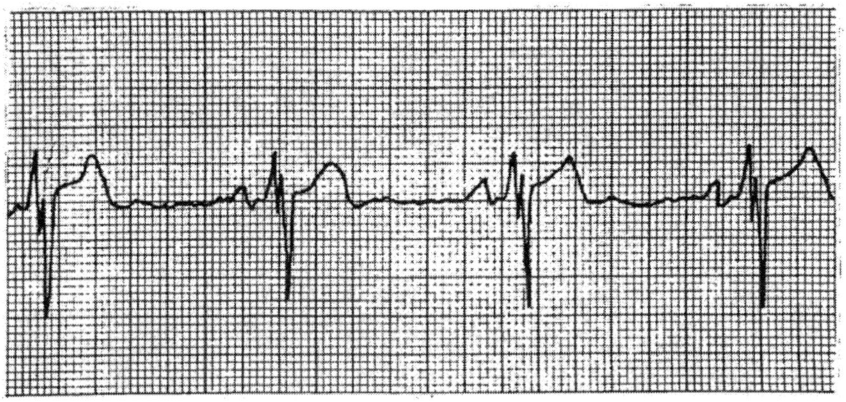

Figure 2-13. Sinus bradycardia.

c. **Sinus Tachycardia.**

(1) Analysis. In sinus tachycardia, the rhythm is regular, the R-R and P-P intervals are constant. Atrial and ventricular rates are equal to or greater than 100 beats per minute. The P wave is normal and upright with one P wave in front of every QRS complex. The P-R interval is constant between 0.12 and 0.20 seconds, and the QRS complex measures less than 0.12 seconds. A variety of circumstances can cause sinus tachycardia: pain, fever, hypoxia, shock, congestive heart failure, and drugs such as epinephrine, atropine, isoproterenol. The more rapid the heart rate, the harder the heart works which can lead to further heart damage in AMI. Also, because there is insufficient time between contractions for the ventricles to fill completely with blood, the heart may not be able to pump fluid effectively when the heart rate is more than 120 to 140 beats per minute. Strenuous exercise such as jogging may cause this condition.

(2) Treatment. Treatment for sinus tachycardia is to treat the cause of this irregularity (fever, fear, blood loss, and so forth.).

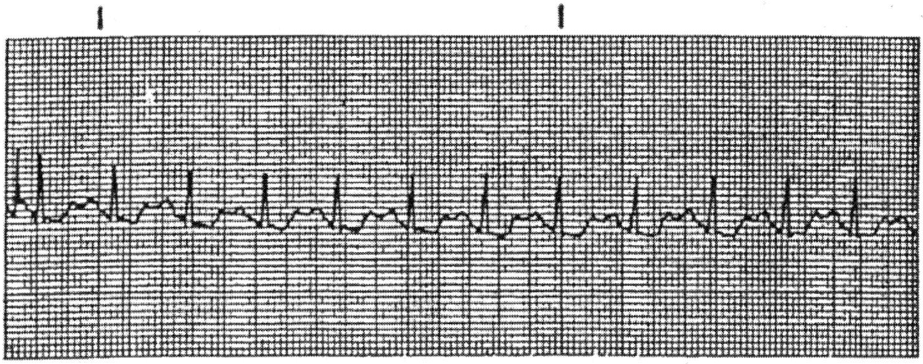

Figure 2-14. Sinus tachycardia. (file: 571f2-14.pcx)

2-8. ATRIAL RHYTHMS

a. **Identification.** The sinus node loses its pacemaking role, and the site with the fastest rate becomes the pacemaker. In this case, the atria is the fastest pacemaker and takes over the pacemaking role. The P wave configuration of atrial rhythms may be flattened, notched, peaked, sawtoothed, diphasic, or upright. The QRS complexes are narrow. Atrial arrhythmia may be caused by irritability of the heart or escape mechanisms of the heart.

NOTE: An escape mechanism is defined as an impulse from somewhere along the conduction pathway that "escapes" to emit an electrical impulse of its own. This electrical impulse stimulates an otherwise electrically quiet heart.

b. **Wandering Pacemaker.**

(1) Analysis. The rhythm is slightly irregular with a normal heartbeat rate of from sixty to one hundred beats per minute. The P wave may change from heartbeat to heartbeat. The PR interval is less than 0.20 of a second and may vary. The QRS is less than 0.12 of a second. If the cardiac output falls, sympathomimetic or parasympatholytic drugs can be given.

(2) Treatment. There is no treatment. The pacemaker shifts between the SA node and the atria. This shift causes each P wave to differ slightly from the P waves around it.

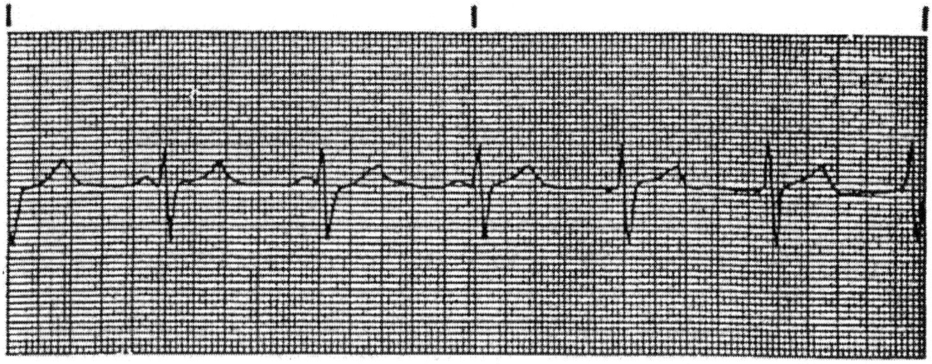

Figure 2-15. Wandering pacemaker.

c. **Premature Atrial Contractions.**

(1) Analysis. Premature Atrial Contractions (PACs) are single heartbeats that originate in the atria and come early in the cardiac cycle. The rhythm depends on the underlying rhythm that will usually be regular except for the premature atrial contraction. The heartbeat rate is usually normal depending on the underlying rhythm. The P waves of the early beat differ from sinus P waves. These P waves can be flattened or notched and thus lost in the preceding T wave. The P-R interval is 0.12 to 0.20 of a second but can be greater than 0.20 of a second. The QRS is less than 0.12 of a second. Isolated PACs may occur in "normal' cardiovascularly healthy people. Frequent PACs may indicate organic heart disease and possibly initiate atrial tachyarrhythmias.

(2) Treatment. The patient should be sedated. Stimulants such as alcohol, caffeine, and tobacco should be eliminated.

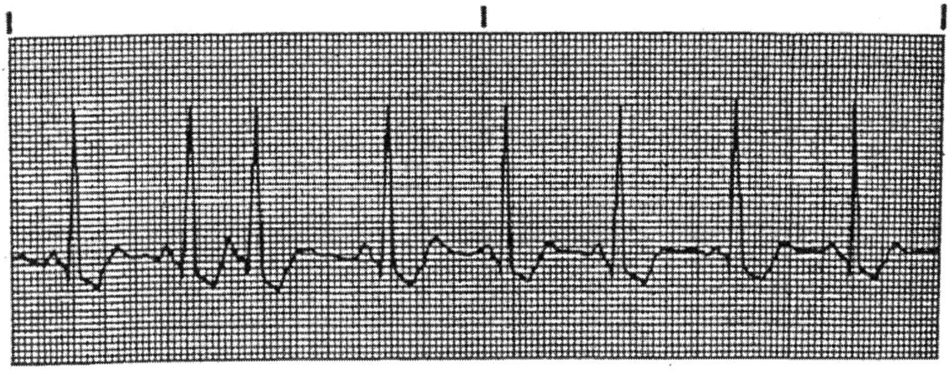

Figure 2-16. Premature atrial contraction (PAC).

d. **Atrial Tachycardia.**

(1) Analysis. Atrial tachycardia (AT) is caused when a single focus in the atria fires very rapidly and overrides the SA node. The rhythm is regular and the heartbeat rate is 150 to 250 beats per minute. The atrial P wave differs from the sinus P wave and can be lost in the preceding T wave. The PR interval is 0.12 to 0.20 of a second with the QRS less than 0.12 of a second. There are two forms of clinical atrial tachycardia: paroxysmal AT/supraventricular tachycardia (PAT/PSVT) and nonparoxysmal AT. Paroxysmal AT/supraventricular tachycardia is characterized by repeated episodes of atrial tachycardia. The episodes may begin abruptly and last from a few seconds to many hours. Nonparoxysmal atrial tachycardia is an abnormal heart problem that is secondary to some other problem.

(2) Treatment. Treatment for nonparoxysmal AT is the same as for sinus tachycardia. See paragraph 2-7c. Treatment for PAT/PSVT is as follows:

(a) Unstable patient (blood pressure less than 90 mm Hg, systolic):

1 Administer synchronized cardioversion of 75 to 100 joules.

2 If there is no response, repeat at 200 joules.

3 If there is still no response, repeat synchronized cardioversion at 360 joules.

4 Correct any underlying abnormalities.

5 Give pharmacological therapy; perform cardioversion.

(b) Stable patient (blood pressure more than 90 mm Hg, systolic):

1 Perform vagal maneuvers.

2 If there is no response, administer verapamil in the dosage of 0.075 to 0.15 mg/kg body weight (maximum 10 mg) as IV bolus over a 1-minute period.

3 If the initial response is not satisfactory and a repeat dose is required, administer at 0.15 mg/kg body weight (maximum 10 mg) 30 minutes after the first dose.

4 If there is still no response, perform cardioversion or use other drug therapy according to a doctor's order.

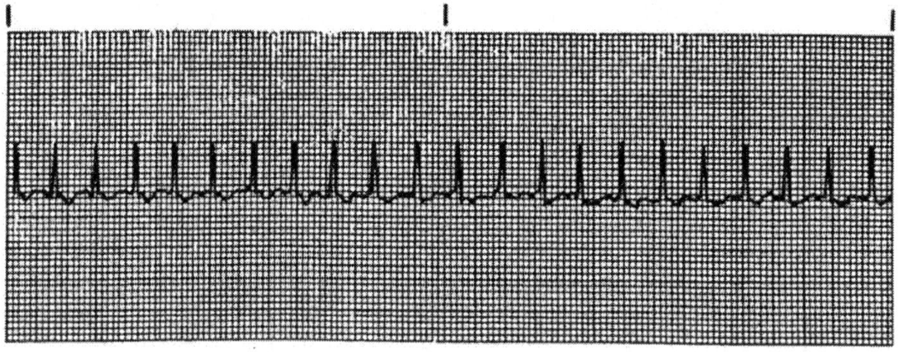

Figure 2-17. Atrial tachycardia.

e. **Atrial Flutter.**

(1) Analysis. Atrial rhythm is regular if the PP intervals are constant. The ventricular rhythm is regular if the AV node conducts impulses in a constant pattern. The ventricular rhythm is irregular if the AV node varies the pattern. In regard to the heartbeat rate, the atrial rate is 250 to 350 heartbeats per minute. The ventricular heartbeat rate depends on the ratio of impulses conducted to the ventricles. The P waves have well defined "flutter" waves and a sawtooth appearance. The P-R interval is not measured (impossible to determine). The QRS complex is less than 0.12 seconds.

(2) Treatment.

(a) There is no treatment if the casualty is hemodynamically (having to do with the movements of the circulation of blood) stable.

(b) If the patient is experiencing a falling blood pressure, cool and clammy skin, confusion, or unconsciousness, treatment is directed at slowing the ventricular rate. In the field, transport the casualty to a medical treatment facility where he can be monitored. DO NOT use cardioversion for a casualty who has been taking digitalis or a person who has a ventricular rate of more than 120 to 140 beats per minute. Cardioversion would not be used if the casualty were experiencing inadequate cardiac output resulting in hypotension, cold and clammy skin, confusion, or coma. Cardioversion would be indicated only when it would be a long time before the casualty could be transported to a medical treatment facility.

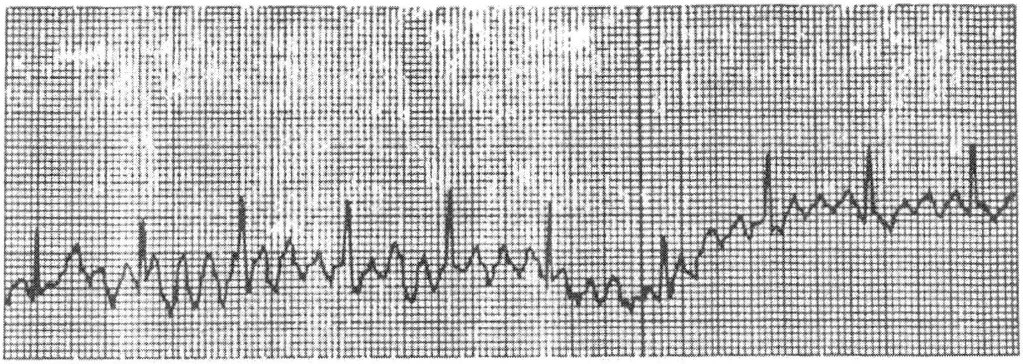

Figure 2-18. Atrial flutter.

f. **Atrial Fibrillation.**

(1) Analysis. In atrial fibrillation, the rhythm is irregularly irregular. The atrial rhythm is unmeasurable, and the R-R interval is irregularly irregular (ventricular). In regard to the heartbeat rate, the atrial rate is unmeasurable. If the ventricular rate is less than 100 beats per minute, it is controlled. If the ventricular rate is greater than 100 beats per minute, it has a rapid ventricular response that is uncontrolled. The atrial heartbeat rate is unmeasurable. The ventricular heartbeat rate, if controlled, is less than 100 beats per minute. If the ventricular heartbeat rate is uncontrolled, the rate is greater than 100 beats per minute. There is either no P wave or there are fibrillatory P waves in which case there is no depolarization of atria, and the waves at the baseline have chaotic undulations. The P-R interval cannot be measured. The QRS complex is less than 0.12 seconds. Atrial fibrillation is usually the result of underlying heart disease. Occasionally, this problem may occur in a normal patient or in patients with MI, especially if SA node infarction occurs. Rapid ventricular response reduces ventricular filling decreasing the stroke volume.

(2) Treatment. Treatment is directed toward eliminating the cause of the problem and decreasing the rate of ventricular response. In the field, transport the casualty to a medical treatment facility and monitor him.

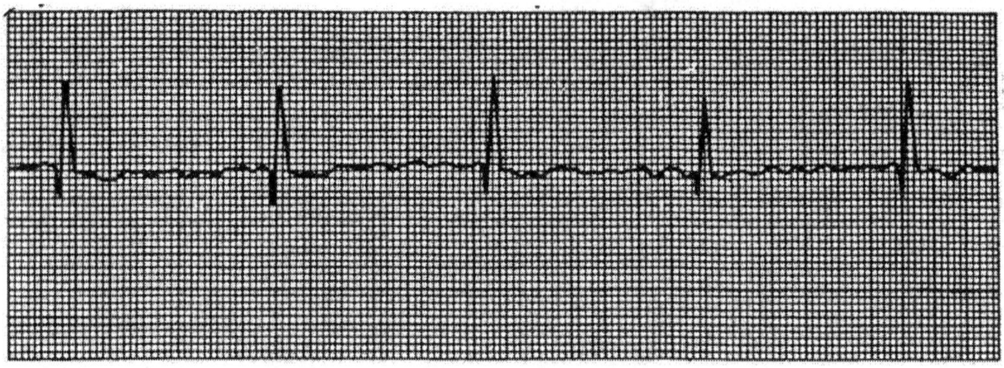

Figure 2-19. Atrial fibrillation (slow).

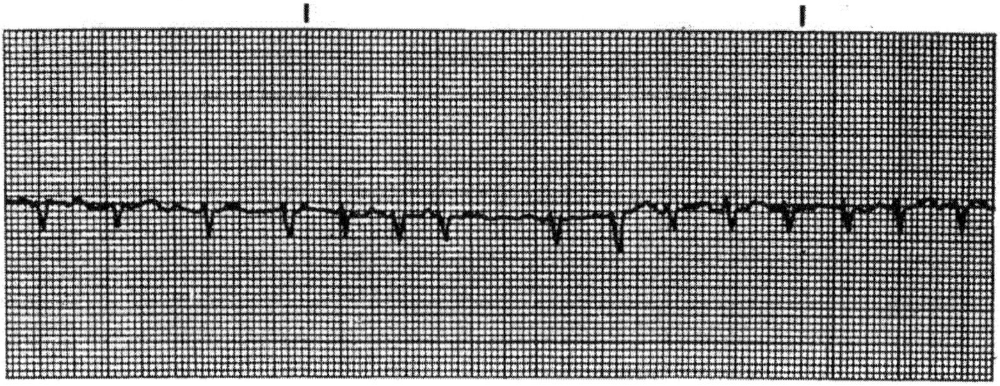

Figure 2-20. Atrial fibrillation (rapid).

2-9. JUNCTIONAL RHYTHMS

a. **General Information.** Junctional arrhythmias create an inverted P wave because the atria are depolarized by the retrograde conduction. These abnormal conditions will depolarize the ventricles in the normal manner (normal QRS). An inverted P wave can occur before, during, or after the QRS complex. All junctional rhythms will create an inverted P wave, but some low atrial impulses can also cause inverted P waves.

b. **Premature Junctional Contraction.**

(1) Analysis. Premature junctional contraction (PJC) is another form of heart abnormality. This condition occurs when a small region of the heart becomes more excitable than normal. This causes an occasional abnormal impulse to be generated between the normal impulses. The abnormal impulse is generated from the region of the heart called the ectopic focus. A wave of depolarization spreads out from the ectopic focus and causes a premature contraction. The regularity depends on the regularity of the underlying rhythm, and the rate depends on the rate of the underlying rhythm. P waves will be inverted and can fall before, during, or after the QRS complex. The PR interval can only be measured if the P wave precedes the QRS Complex. The QRS complex lasts less than 0.12 of a second. What happens is that the AV node takes over the pacemaking function.

(2) Treatment. Treatment is the same as for premature atrial contractions (PACs). See paragraph 2-8c.

NOTE: The normal inherent rate of atrial ventricular junction is 40 to 60 beats per minute. If higher pacemaker sites fail, a junctional escape pacemaker might take control of the heart. The rhythm would then be called a junctional escape rhythm. Inherent rates are as follows: atria--75 beats/minute; A-V node - 60 beats/minute; ventricles--40 to 60 beats per minute; and normal heart rate - 60 to 100 beats per minute.

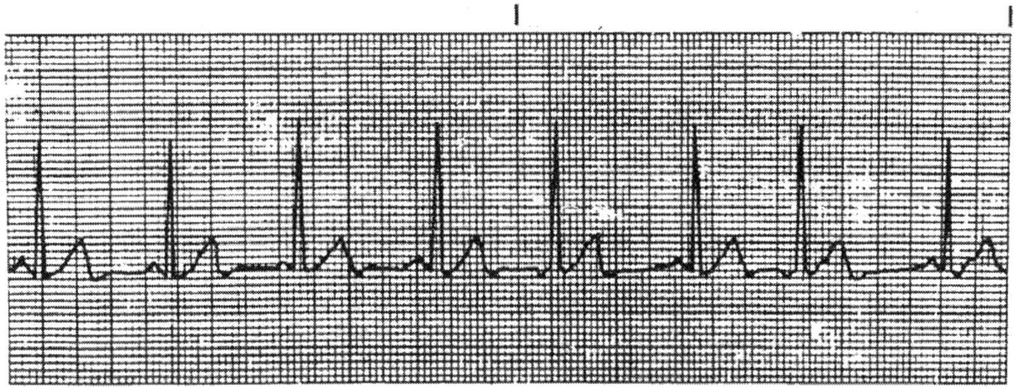

Figure 2-21. Premature junctional contractions (PJC).

2-10. **HEART BLOCKS**

a. **General Information.** Heart blocks are arrhythmias caused by conduction disturbances at the AV node.

b. **First-Degree (Incomplete) Heart Block.**

(1) Analysis. The first-degree heart block takes place where there is an incomplete block. The regularity and rate depend on the underlying rhythm of the heart. The P waves are upright and uniform and followed by the QRS complex. The PR interval is constant and greater than 0.20 seconds. The QRS complex is less than 0.12 seconds.

(2) Treatment. There is no treatment.

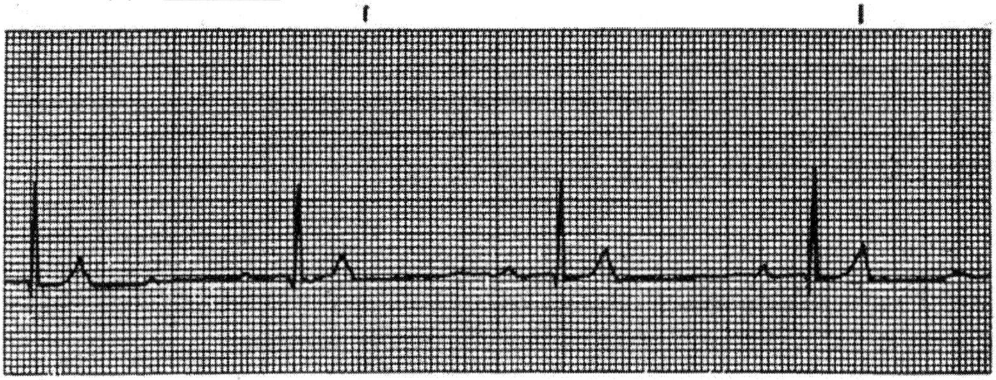

Figure 2-22. First degree (incomplete) heart block.

c. **Wenckebach (Second-Degree Heart Block/Mobitz Type 1).**

(1) Analysis. The rhythm is irregular, and the R-R interval gets progressively shorter as the P-R intervals get longer. Grouped beating is characteristic. The heartbeat rate is usually slightly slower than normal. P waves are upright and uniform, but some P waves are not followed by QRS complexes. The P-R interval progressively lengthens until one P wave is not conducted. The QRS complex lasts less than 0.12 of a second. This condition is a less serious type of second-degree heart block. It is, however, still quite common in patients with acute myocardial infarction. The condition may be produced by digitalis.

(2) Treatment. The casualty should be transported to a medical treatment facility and monitored. If the heart rate is very slow, give atropine in the dosage 0.5 mg every five minutes to a total dose of 2.0 mg intravenously or until the heartbeat rate is up to 60 beats per minute.

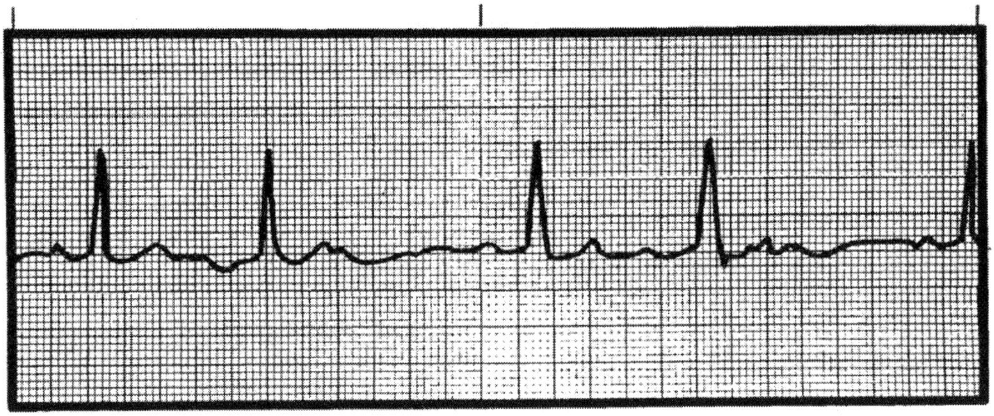

Figure 2-23. Wenckebach (second-degree heart block/Mobitz Type I).

d. **Classical Second-Degree Heart Block (Mobitz Type II).**

(1) Analysis. The rhythm is regular if the conduction ratio is constant; however, the rhythm is irregular if the conduction ratio varies. The rate for atrial is usually normal, and the ventricular rate is usually bradycardia. P waves are upright and uniform with more P waves than QRS complexes (usually a ratio of 2:1, 3:1, and so forth.). The P-R interval is constant on conducted beats, but it may be longer than normal.

(2) Treatment. If the cardiac output is adequate, there is no treatment. If there are signs of an inadequate cardiac output, treat with 0.5 mg atropine sulfate IV bolus. This dose may be repeated until the pulse reaches 60 or more beats per minute or until a maximum dose of 2.0 mg has been given. If atropine sulfate is ineffective, administer 2 mg of isoproteronal in 500 cc D5W IV piggyback until the blood pressure is 80 or the heart rate is greater than 60. Radio the medical treatment facility to have a pacemaker ready.

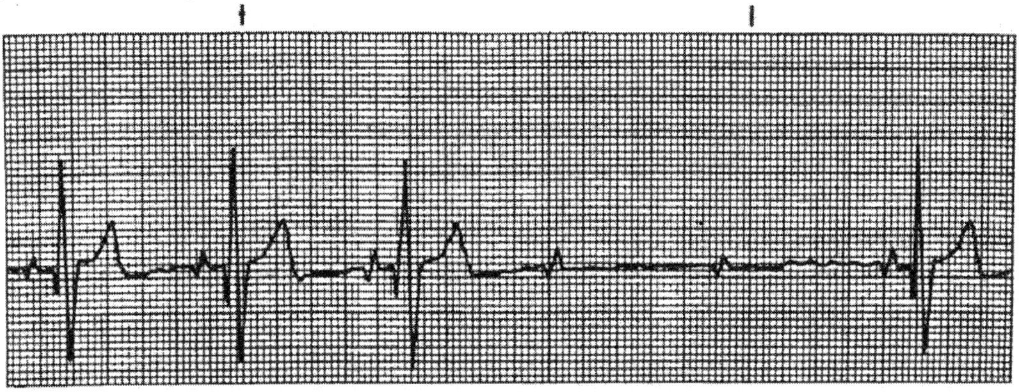

Figure 2-24. Classical second-degree heart block (Mobitz Type II).

e. **Complete Heart Block (Third-Degree).**

(1) Analysis. The rhythm is regular with PP and RR intervals constant. The atrial rate is normal, but the ventrical response rate varies in this way. The junction focus has a rate of 40 to 60 beats per minute. The ventrical focus has a rate of 20 to 40 beats per minute. P waves are upright and uniform with more P waves than QRS complexes. There are no PR intervals because the P waves have no relationship to QRS complexes. Occasionally, a P wave is superimposed on a QRS complex. The QRS complex is less than 0.12 seconds at the junctional focus and greater than 0.12 seconds at the ventricular focus. Cardiac output may be greatly diminished if the heart rate is below 35 to 50 beats per minute. Additionally, in third-degree heart block, the atria and ventricles are no longer synchronized; therefore, the ventricles do not fill completely before each contraction, causing cardiac output to be even further reduced. The ventricular rate may be so slow that circulation cannot be maintained and syncope (congestive heart failure) or angina may occur.

(2) Treatment. Administer atropine sulfate 0.5 mg IV bolus and repeat at 5-minute intervals to try to maintain a heart rate greater than 60 or until the maximum dose of 2.0 mg is given. If this treatment is ineffective, administer isoproteronal 2 mg in 500 cc D5W IV piggyback until the blood pressure is 80 or the heart rate is greater than 60. NEVER give lidocaine to a casualty with complete heart block. Lidocaine may increase the threshold of the conduction system and block part of the conduction pathways. (You must be able to tell the difference between PVCs and complete heart block.) And, finally, radio a doctor to have a pacemaker ready.

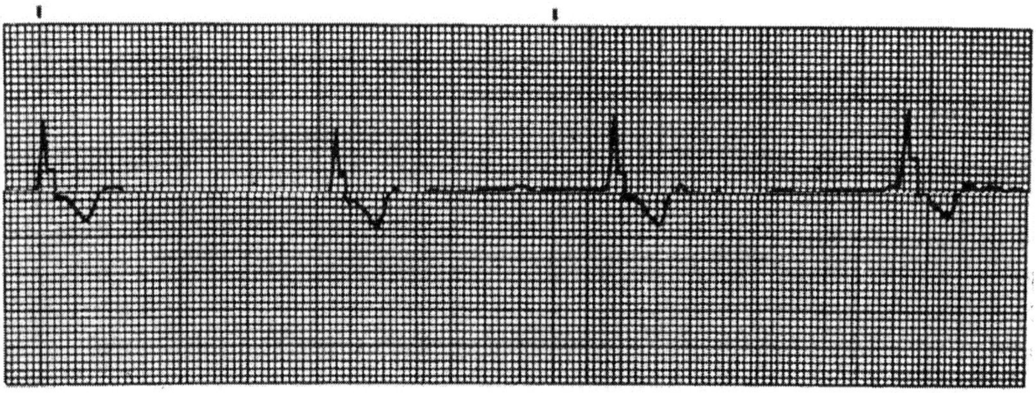

Figure 2-25. Complete heart block.

2-11. **VENTRICULAR ARRHYTHMIAS.**

a. **General.** Ventricular arrhythmias are the most serious arrhythmias. The definition of arrhythmia is an abnormality in the rate, rhythm, or conduction of the heartbeat. A heartbeat irregularity may be an indication of some disease or a normal response to the body's activity. Arrhythmias are classified on the basis of the site of origin of the arrhythmia: SA node, atria, AV node, or ventricle. As with some heart blocks, the QRS complex measurement is equal to or greater than 0.12 seconds. A QRS of less than 0.12 of a second indicates a supraventricular pacemaker. If the QRS is 0.12 of a second or greater, the problem could be ventricular or supraventricular with ventricular conduction defect. All ventricular arrhythmias will have a QRS complex of 0.12 of a second or greater. The reason ventricular rhythms are the most serious arrhythmias is that the heart is less effective than usual and is functioning on its last level of backup support. Four types of ventricular arrhythmias will be covered here: premature ventricular contractions, ventricular tachycardia, ventricular fibrillation, and idioventricular rhythm.

b. **Premature Ventricular Contractions.**

(1) Analysis. A premature ventricular contractions (PVCs) is a single ectopic (heartbeat arising from a place other than the SA node) caused by irritable focus in the ventricles. The heartbeat comes earlier than expected and interrupts the regularity of the underlying rhythm of the heart. The heartbeat rate is determined by the underlying heartbeat rhythm, PVCs not being included in the rate. P waves will not come before an ectopic heartbeat; however, P waves may be seen near a premature ventricular contraction. Since the heartbeat comes from a lower focus, there will be no P-R interval. The QRS complex will be wide and bizarre (at least 0.12 or more of a second). The T wave is usually in the opposite direction from the R wave. Premature ventricular contractions may be quite serious, particularly in certain combinations and in the wake of acute myocardial infarction. Dangerous signs include frequent PVCs, runs of PVCs, multifocal PVCs, and the R-on-T phenomenon. In a perfectly healthy person, PVCs may not always be considered an abnormality; however, if the casualty is experiencing acute myocardial infarction, PVCs must be treated instantly.

(2) Characteristics. The following are characteristic of premature ventricular contractions:

(a) A compensatory pause usually follows a PVC. The distance between the R wave of complex preceding the PVC and the R wave of complex following the PVC is exactly twice the R-R interval of underlying rhythm.

(b) The PVC does not have to have a compensatory pause. The beat can be "interpolated" between two sinus beats without interrupting the underlying rhythm.

(c) Premature ventricular contractions indicate myocardial irritability. The frequency of PVCs suggests the degree of myocardial irritability.

(d) Premature ventricular contractions are considered <u>unifocal</u> if they all originate from a single ventricular focus and have similar configurations.

(e) Premature ventricular contractions are considered <u>multifocal</u> if they original from many different points and have different configurations.

(f) If a PVC occurs during a vulnerable (relative refractory) phase of the cardiac cycle, the PVC can produce lethal, repetitive arrhythmias. A PVC that falls on the downslope of a T wave is referred to as "R-on-T" phenomenon and is considered very dangerous.

(g) With increasing irritability, PVCs can occur in pairs called couplets or in runs of three or more consecutive ectopics (ectopic heartbeat originating from a place other than the SA node).

(h) Premature ventricular contractions frequently occur in patterns such as the following:

<u>1</u> Bigeminy--a PVC every other heartbeat.

<u>2</u> Trigeminy--a PVC every third beat.

<u>3</u> Quadrigeminy--a PVC every fourth beat.

NOTE: Bigeminy, trigeminy, and quadrigeminy can also describe patterns of premature atrial contractions (PACS) and premature junctional contractions (PJCs).

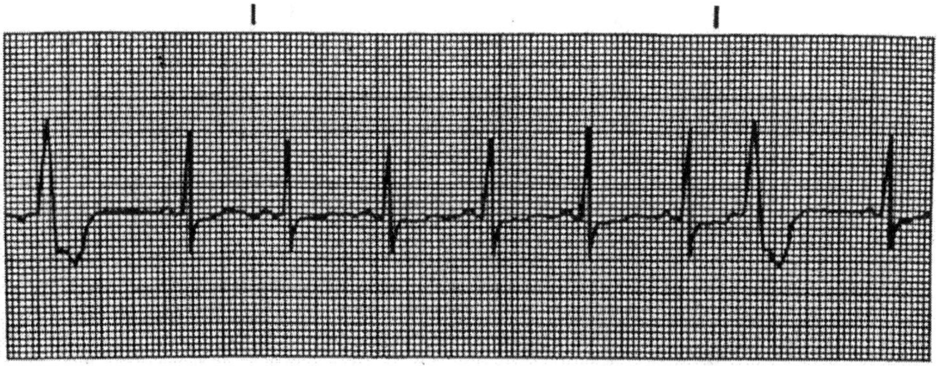

Figure 2-26. Frequent premature ventricular contractions.

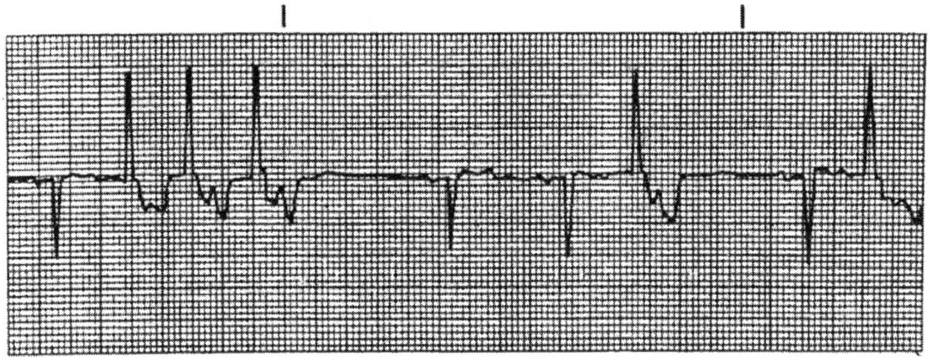

Figure 2-27. Runs of premature ventricular contractions.

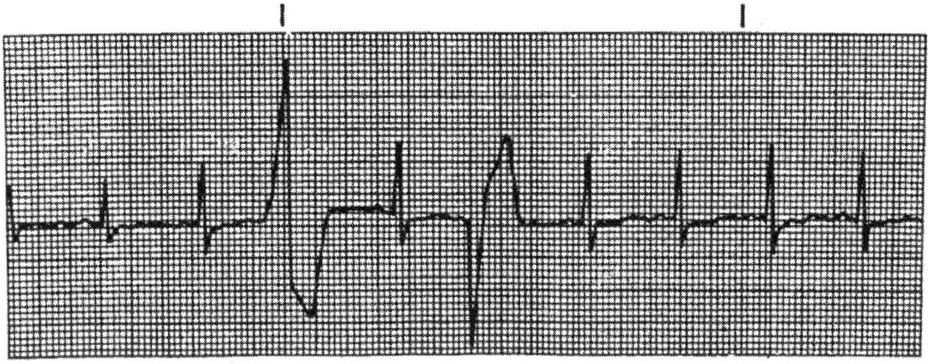

Figure 2-28. Multifocal premature ventricular contractions.

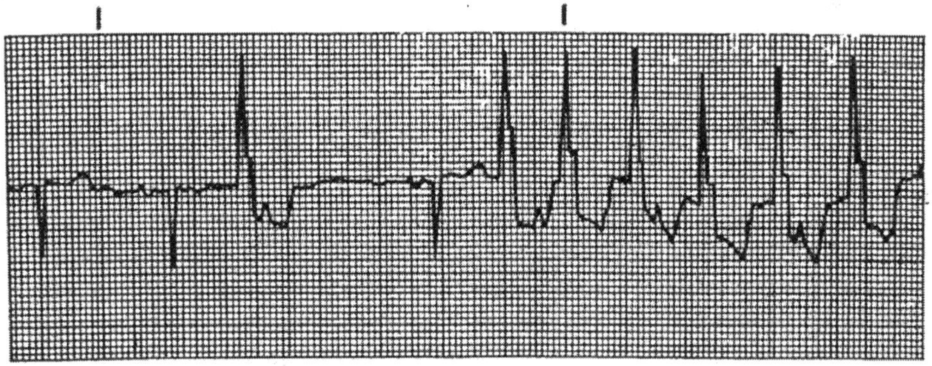

Figure 2-29. Runs of premature ventricular contractions with short run of ventricular tachycardia.

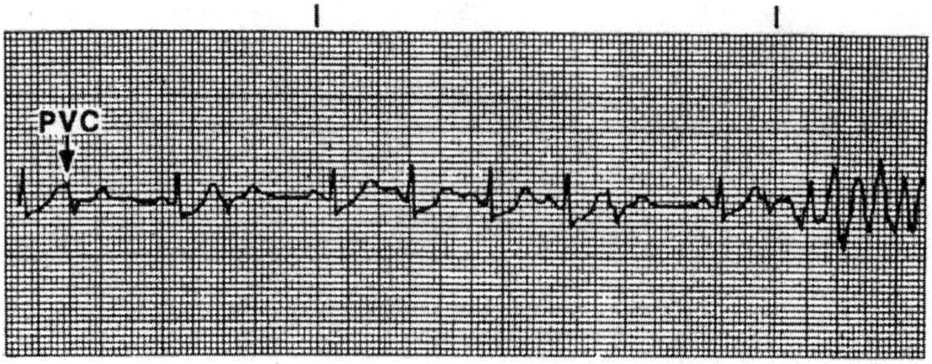

Figure 2-30. R-on-T phenomenon ending in ventricular fibrillation.

(3) Treatment. Administer lidocaine.

(a) Administer lidocaine if any or all of the following are present:

1 Frequent PVCs (more than 6 per minute).

2 Premature ventricular contractions frequently coupled.

3 Multifocal PVCs (Premature ventricular contractions which are different shapes and sizes).

4 Bursts of two or more PVCs in succession.

(b) Give this dosage:

1 Initially, give 1.0 mg per kilogram of weight of lidocaine IV bolus.

2 Additionally, 0.5 mg/kg IV boluses can be given every 2 to 10 minutes, if necessary to a total of 3 mg/kg intravenously.

(c) If transport time is excessive, consider continuous infusion at 1 to 4 mg/minute.

(d) If PVCs occur and the casualty is also experiencing bradycardia, treat the bradycardia first.

c. **Ventricular Tachycardia.**

(1) Analysis. The rhythm of the heart is usually regular, but the rhythm can be slightly irregular. The heartbeat rate is from 150 to 250 beats per minute. The rate can exceed 250 beats per minute of the heart rhythm progressing to ventricular flutter. Occasionally, the rate may be slower than 150 beats per minute; the condition is then termed slow ventricular tachycardia (VT). P waves are not normally seen; however, dissociated waves may be seen. The focus is in the ventricles, and there will be no PR interval. The QRS complex is wide and bizarre. The complex may be 0.12 of a second or greater. The T wave is usually in the opposite direction from the R wave. Ventricular tachycardia is serious and dangerous. It may be the precursor of ventricular fibrillation. If VT persists, there may be a marked reduction in cardiac output.

(2) Treatment. Begin with lidocaine intravenously unless the situation is critical, then give a DC countershock.

NOTE: If the casualty has no pulse, treat as you would for ventricular fibrillation. Treatment for a stable and unstable casualty is not the same.

(a) Stable casualty. Follow this procedure for the casualty who has no symptoms (no chest pain or dyspnea, adequate blood pressure, and a pulse):

1 Administer lidocaine 1 mg/kg intravenously bolus. This may be followed by 0.5 mg/kg intravenously every 8 minutes until the ventricular tachycardia resolves or up to 3 mg/kg intravenously.

2 Give procainamide 2 mg/minute intra-venously until the ventricular tachycardia resolves or up to 1,000 mg intravenously. (Use procainamide if lidocaine doesn't work.)

3 If drug therapy is not successful, perform low energy cardioversion of 50 joules.

4 If a defibrillator is available, use a mechanical means of conversions ("chest thump" or "cough.")

NOTE: Mechanical conversion may cause ventricular fibrillation.

(b) Unstable casualty. Follow this procedure for the casualty who has chest pain, a systolic blood pressure less than 90 mm Hg, and a pulse.

1 Perform nonsynchronized cardioversion in the following sequence:

a Give 50 joules.

b If there is no change, give 100 joules.

c If there is still no change, give 200 joules.

d If there is still no change, give 360 joules.

2 Administer lidocaine 1 mg/kg intra-venously bolus. This may be followed by 0.5 mg/kg intravenously every 8 minutes up to a total of 3 mg/kg intravenously.

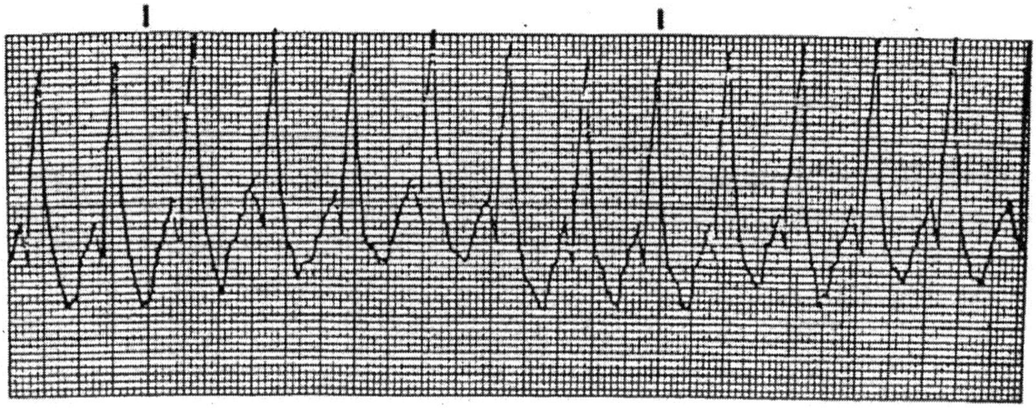

Figure 2-31. Ventricular tachycardia.

d. **Ventricular Fibrillation).**

(1) Analysis. The rhythm, rate, P waves, P-R interval, and QRS complex are totally chaotic with no discernible waves or complete complexes in this abnormality. The ventricles fire in a totally disorganized fashion, and, instead of beating, the ventricular muscle quivers. Consequently, there is no cardiac output, and the ventricular fibrillation is the same as death. The casualty is clinically dead. Normal heart rhythm must be restored within a few minutes or biologic death follows. When you see a rhythm on the monitor that resembles ventricular fibrillation, check quickly to be sure this pattern is not caused by muscle tremor, loose leads, or patient movement artifact.

(2) Treatment. For a witnessed arrest, first check the patient for a pulse. I there is no pulse, perform a precordial thump. Again check for a pulse; if there is no pulse, perform CPR until a defibrillator is available. For an unwitnessed arrest, check for a pulse. If there is no pulse, perform CPR until a defibrillator is available. Follow this procedure for either a witnessed arrest or an unwitnessed arrest once a monitor is available:

(a) Check the monitor for rhythm.

(b) Defibrillate at 200 joules. Check the pulse and rhythm.

(c) If this is unsuccessful, defibrillate at 200 to 300 joules. (Again, if VF recurs, use the energy level previously successful.)

(d) If still unsuccessful, defibrillate up to 360 joules.

(e) If there is no pulse, perform CPR.

(f) Establish IV access.

(g) Administer epinephrine, 1:10,000, 0.5 - 1.0 mg IV Push. (Repeat epinephrine every 5 minutes.)

(h) Intubate, if possible.

(i) Administer lidocaine, 1 mg/kg IV Push.

(j) Defibrillate with up to 360 joules. (Again, if VF occurs, defibrillate with the energy level previously successful.)

(k) Administer bretylium, 5 mg/kg IV Push.

(l) Consider bicarbonate.

(m) Defibrillate with up to 360 joules. (If VP recurs, defibrillate with the energy level previously successful.)

(n) Administer bretylium, 10 mg/kg IV Push.

(o) Defibrillate with up to 360 joules. (If VF recurs, defibrillate with the energy level previously successful.)

(p) Administer either lidocaine or bretylium.

(q) Defibrillate with up to 360 joules. (If VF recurs, defibrillate with the energy level previously successful.)

NOTE: This sequence of treatment is appropriate for a broad range of patients. It may be necessary to make some changes in treatment in individual cases.

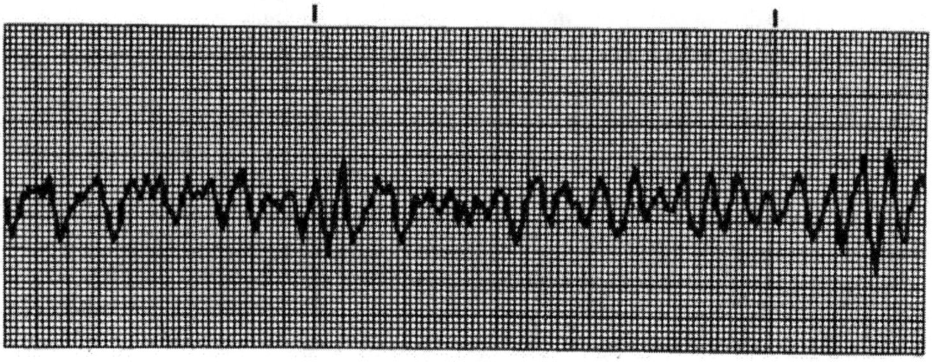

Figure 2-32. Ventricular fibrillation (fine).

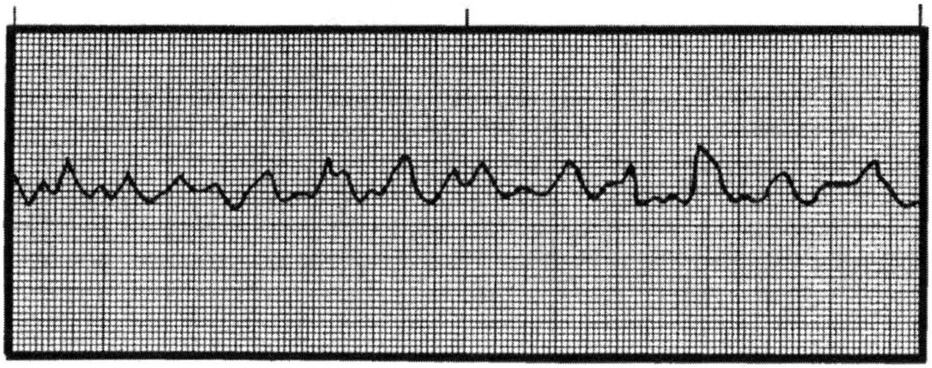

Figure 2-33. Ventricular fibrillation (coarse).

e. **Idioventricular Rhythm.**

(1) Analysis. The rhythm is usually regular, but can be unreliable, since the rhythm of the heart is at such a low site. There is no P wave nor P-R interval. The QRS complex is wide and bizarre and 0.12 second or greater. The escape rhythm has taken over the pacemaking responsibility.

(2) Treatment. Treat as follows:

(a) First administer atropine.

(b) If atropine is unsuccessful, administer isoprel.

(c) If there is no improvement, perform a fluid challenge. Administer 500 cc IV fluid quickly until the patient has received two liters of fluid.

(d) In a hospital setting, if the patient's condition has not improved, an internal or external pacemaker is considered.

(e) If there is still no improvement, the next step is chest massage.

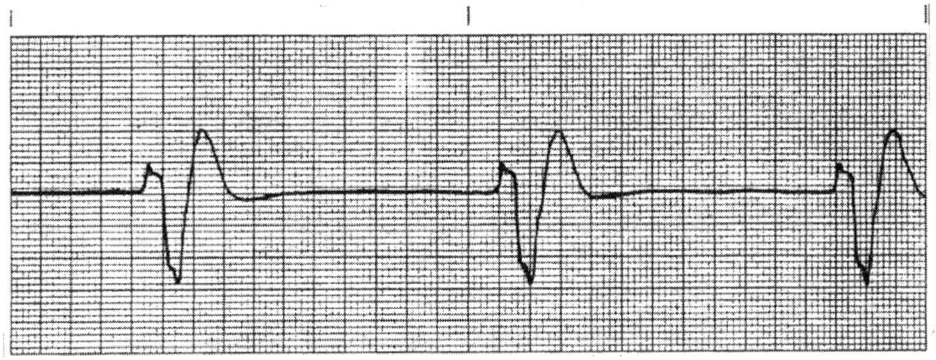

Figure 2-34. Idioventricular rhythm.

2-12. **ASYSTOLE (CARDIAC STANDSTILL)**

a. **Analysis.** A straight line on the electrocardiogram indicates an absence of electrical activity by the heart: no regularity, rate, P waves, P-R interval, or QRS complex. The casualty is clinically dead. He has no effective cardiac output. Normal rhythm must be restored within a few minutes by appropriate treatment.

b. **Treatment.** It is sometimes difficult to distinguish between asystole and ventricular fibrillation. If there is any doubt, treat the patient for ventricular fibrillation. When the rhythm is unclear and the possibility of VT exists, defibrillate as for ventricular fibrillation. If asystole is present, follow this procedure:

(1) Continue CPR.

(2) Establish IV access.

(3) Administer epinephrine, 1:10,000, 0.5 - 1.0 mg IV push.

(4) Intubate when possible.

(5) Administer atropine, 1.0 mg IV push, repeated in 5 minutes.

(6) Consider bicarbonate.

(7) Consider pacing (the use of an internal or external pacemaker).

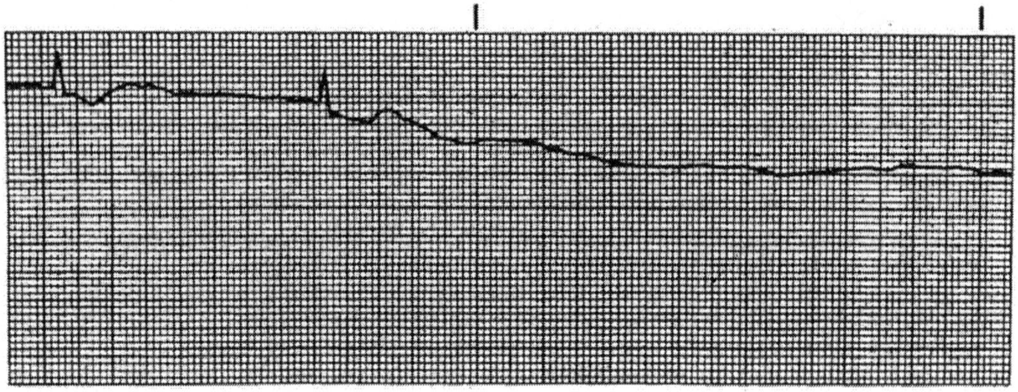

Figure 2-35. Asystole (cardiac standstill).

Continue with Exercises

EXERCISES, LESSON 2

INSTRUCTIONS: The following exercises are to be answered by writing the answer in the space provided. After you have completed all the exercises, turn to "Solutions to Exercises" at the end of the lesson and check your answers.

1. When you are calculating regular rhythms, the most accurate method is to count the number of small squares between ____________________ and divide that number into 1500.

2. The rate for irregular rhythm is based on the ______________ strip method.

3. In atrial polarization, the P waves seen on the oscilloscope indicate __________________________________ deflections.
   (small or large) (positive or negative)

4. Q waves occurring on the oscilloscope are ____________________ deflections.

5. The rhythm for sinus bradycardia is ___________________with the PR intervals ___________________ and the PP intervals ___________________________.

6. Administer ______________ when you treat sinus bradycardia with hypotension.

7. The casualty's heartbeat rhythm is regular (RRI and PPI are constant). The atrial and ventricular waves are equal to or greater than 100 beats per minute. The P wave is uniform with one P wave appearing in front of every QRS complex. The P-R interval is constant between 0.12 and 0.20 seconds. The QRS measures less than 0.12 seconds. Which cardiac dysrhythmia is the casualty suffering from?

   ____

8. A soldier in the field is experiencing atrial fibrillation. His pulse is rapid. Treatment is to ______________________________________and monitor him.

9. In the dysrhythmia, ______________________________ the rhythm is regular, the RR and PP intervals are constant, and the atrial and ventricular rates are equal to or greater than 100 beats per minute.

10. In the case of atrial rhythms, the sinus node loses its pacemaking role, and the site with the ______________________________ becomes the pacemaker.

11. What is the treatment for wandering pacemaker atrial rhythm?

____.

12. A single focus in the atria fires very rapidly and overrides the SA node. The name of this atrial rhythm is ______________________________.

13. Premature junctional contraction (PJC) occurs when a small region of the heart becomes ______________________________.

14. What is the general cause of heart blocks? ______________________________

15. A premature ventricular contraction (PVC) is a single ectopic heartbeat which comes earlier than expected ______________________________ and the regularity of the underlying rhythm of the heart.

16. A characteristic of ventricular fibrillation (VF) is that the ventricles of the heart fire in a ______________ instead of beating, the ventricular muscle ______________.

17. Another name for cardiac standstill is ______________________________.

18. List five atrial rhythms dealt with in this lesson.

a. ______________________________________.

b. ______________________________________.

c. ______________________________________.

d. ______________________________________.

e. ______________________________________.

19. List four ventricular arrhythmias written about in this lesson.

a. ______________________________________.

b. ______________________________________.

c. ______________________________________.

d. ______________________________________.

20. The one junctional rhythm listed in this lesson is ________________________.

Check Your Answers on Next Page

SOLUTIONS TO EXERCISES, LESSON 2

1. Two R waves. (para 2-6b(l)(a))

2. Six second. (para 2-6b(2))

3. Small. Positive. (para 2-5c(l))

4. Negative. (para 2-5d(2))

5. Regular. Constant. Constant. (para 2-7b(l)(a))

6. Atropine. (para 2-7b(2)(b))

7. Sinus tachycardia. (para 2-7c(l))

8. Transport him to a medical treatment facility. (para 2-8f(2))

9. Sinus tachycardia. (para 2-7c(l))

10. Fastest rate. (para 2-8a)

11. There is no treatment. (para 2-8b(2))

12. Atrial tachycardia (AT). (para 2-8d(l))

13. More excitable than nominal. (para 2-9b(l))

14. Conduction disturbances at the AV node are a general cause of heart blocks. (para 2-10a)

15. Interrupts. (para 2-11b(1)

16. Totally disorganized. Quivers. (para 2-11d(1))

17. Asystole. (para 2-12)

18. Wandering pacemaker.
Premature atrial contractions (PACs).
Atrial tachycardia.
Atrial flutter.
Atrial fibrillation. (paras 2-8b through f)

19. Premature ventricular contractions (PVCs).
    Ventricular tachycardia (VT).
    Ventricular fibrillation (VF).
    Idioventricular rhythm. (paras 2-11b through e)

20. Premature junctional contraction (PJC). (para 2-9(b)

End of Lesson 2

LESSON ASSIGNMENT

LESSON 3	Cardiac Arrest (Defibrillation)
LESSON ASSIGNMENT	Paragraphs 3-1 through 3-15.
LESSON OBJECTIVE	After completing this lesson, you should be able to:
	3-1. Identify the causes, signs, risk factors, and major management techniques of cardiac arrest.
SUGGESTION	After completing the assignment, complete the exercises of this lesson. These exercises will help you to achieve the lesson objectives.

LESSON 3

CARDIAC ARREST (DEFIBRILLATION)

Section I. REVIEW OF THE CARDIOVASCULAR SYSTEM AND THE RESPIRATORY SYSTEM

3-1. DEFINITIONS

Some of the terms used in this and following lessons are defined below.

a. **Casualty.** The casualty is the person with the medical problem, such as a person who is not breathing.

b. **Rescuer.** The rescuer is the person who is assisting the casualty; for example, the person who is giving mouth-to- mouth resuscitation to the casualty.

c. **Airway.** The airway consists of the body structures through which air from the atmosphere passes while going to the lungs. The airway includes the oral and nasal cavities (mouth and nose), pharynx (throat), larynx (voice box), trachea (windpipe), and bronchi (two tubes leading from the trachea to the lungs).

d. **Sign.** A sign is anything that the rescuer can tell about the casualty's condition by using his own senses. For example, a rescuer can <u>see</u> a wound, <u>hear</u> breathing difficulty, <u>feel</u> that the casualty has a fever by touching the casualty's skin, and <u>smell</u> an unusual odor on the casualty's Is breath, a possible sign of poisoning.

e. **Symptom.** A symptom is any change from the norm which is felt by the casualty but which cannot be directly or objectively sensed by the rescuer. Examples of symptoms felt by the victim are chest pains, nausea, a headache, and mental confusion. An injury can produce both signs and symptoms; for example, pain which only the victim can feel and a bump or bruise which can be viewed by others.

f. **Aggravate.** To aggravate a wound means to make it worse. For example, moving a person with a fractured leg before the leg is splinted can cause the sharp ends of the broken bone to cut nerves and blood vessels that were not damaged before the person was moved.

3-2. IMPORTANCE OF FOOD, OXYGEN, AND THE CARDIOVASCULAR SYSTEM

The human body is composed of cells. The average adult's body is made up of around eighty trillion (80,000,000,000,000) living cells. Each living cell needs energy to survive. Cells obtain energy through oxidation. That is, they combine a source of potential energy with oxygen to liberate energy. The sources of potential energy come from the food (carbohydrates, fats, and proteins) that is processed into usable units by the body's digestive system (stomach, small intestines, liver, pancreas, etc.). Oxygen comes from the air that is breathed in and absorbed by the lungs. Oxygen in the lungs and food in the intestines, however, cannot help muscles and other cells unless the oxygen and food can be delivered to those cells. Delivering food and oxygen to the cells is the function of blood and of the body's cardiovascular system.

3-3. THE CARDIOVASCULAR SYSTEM

The cardiovascular system consists of the heart and the blood vessels. The cardiovascular system keeps all parts of the body supplied with blood. Blood brings oxygen and nutrients to the cells and carries away waste products.

a. **Heart.** The heart (figure 3-1) is the pump that keeps the blood circulating. Actually, the heart could be described as two pumps, both of which are under the control of a natural pacemaker called the sinoatrial node. Each side (right half and left half) of the heart has a receiving chamber for the blood called the atrium and a pumping chamber called the ventricle. The two halves of the heart are separated by a wall-like structure called the interventricular septum. The sinoatrial node (SA node), located at the junction of the superior vena cava and the right atrium, is a small bundle of nerve tissue that produces an electrical stimulus. This electrical stimulus causes the muscles of the ventricles to contract.

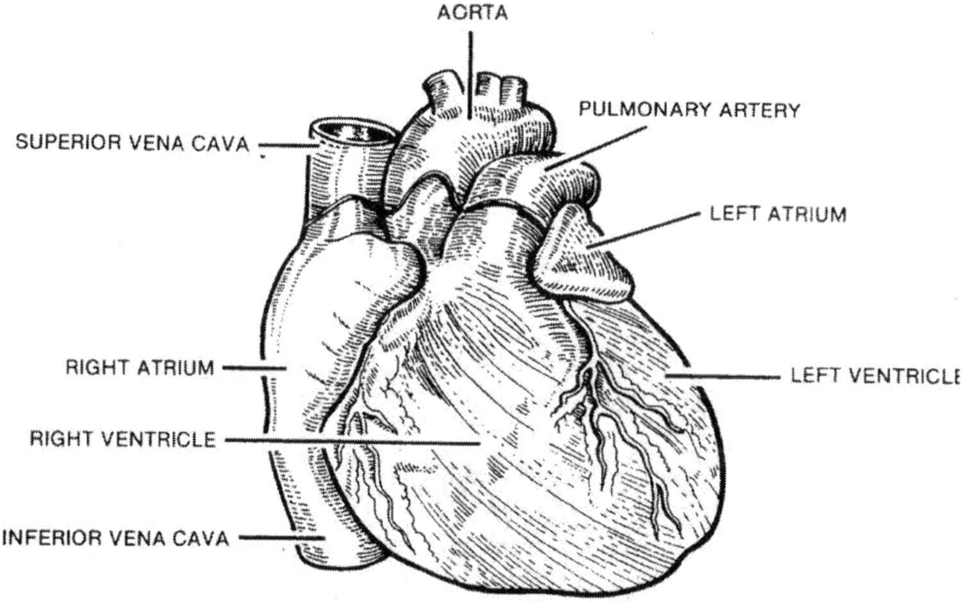

Figure 3-1. The human heart (front view).

b. **Blood Vessels.** The blood vessels of the cardiovascular system carry the blood away from the heart and back to the heart again.

(1) Blood circulation systems. Since the heart is divided into two parts (the right half consisting of the right atrium and the right ventricle and the left half consisting of the left atrium and the left ventricle), it is not surprising to find that there are actually two blood circulatory systems--the systemic and the pulmonary.

(a) Systemic. The systemic (general) circulatory system is the larger of the two systems. It takes the blood pumped by the left ventricle to all parts of the body and returns the blood to the right atrium. The blood is rich in oxygen when it leaves the heart through the left ventricle and is low in oxygen content when it returns to the right atrium.

(b) Pulmonary. The pulmonary circulatory system takes the blood pumped by the right ventricle to the lungs and returns the blood to the left atrium. The blood is oxygen-poor when it leaves the right ventricle and oxygen-rich when it returns to the left atrium.

(2) Types of blood vessels. Both the systemic and the pulmonary circulatory systems are composed of three major types of blood vessels: arteries, capillaries, and veins.

(a) Arteries. Arteries carry blood pumped by the ventricles away from the heart. The arteries of the systemic circulatory system carry oxygenated (oxygen-rich) blood to body tissues. Pulmonary arteries carry deoxygenated (oxygen-poor) blood to the lungs. Arteries have the capacity to constrict and dilate. This constricting and dilating helps regulate blood pressure.

(b) Capillaries. The arteries are large blood vessels that divide into smaller branches. These branches then divide again and again. Each time, the blood vessels become smaller and smaller. Finally, the blood vessels are so small that only one red blood cell can pass through at a time. When they reach this size, the blood vessels are called capillaries. When a blood cell enters the capillaries, it is free to perform its primary functions. In the pulmonary system, the red blood cells give up carbon dioxide to the lungs and pick up oxygen. In the systemic system, blood gives oxygen, nutrients, and fluids to the cells and picks up carbon dioxide and other waste materials.

(c) Veins. Capillaries join together to form larger blood vessels. These blood vessels combine to form even larger blood vessels. This process continues until large blood vessels called veins are formed. Veins carry blood back to the heart. The veins of the systemic system carry oxygen-poor blood to the right atrium. The veins of the pulmonary system carry oxygen-rich blood to the left atrium.

3-4. **THE RESPIRATORY SYSTEM**

The respiratory system consists of two lungs and the respiratory tract that carries air to and from the lungs (figure 3-2). When a person inhales, air enters the nose or mouth, travels down the trachea, and into one of the two bronchi. These air tubes divide into smaller and smaller tubes. Finally, the air reaches the tiny alveoli. These alveoli are like tiny sacs. When air enters an alveolus, the capillaries surrounding the alveolus absorb oxygen and give off carbon dioxide. When a person exhales, the air carrying the carbon dioxide travels from the alveoli through the air tubes, up the trachea, and out of the nose or mouth. Of course, not all of the air inhaled reaches the alveoli nor is all of the oxygen removed from the air in the alveoli. The average adult takes in about 500 milliliters of air each time he inhales, and he exhales the same amount. Even after the person exhales, the lungs still contain about 2300 milliliters of air.

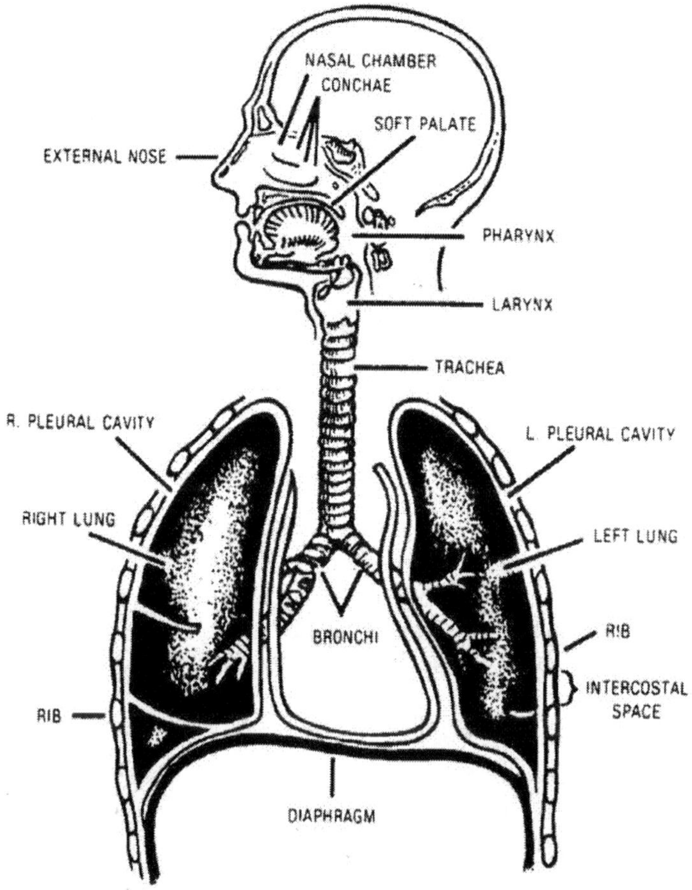

Figure 3-2. The respiratory system.

3-5. **BLOOD FLOW**

In order to summarize how blood flows in the body, let's take a trip through the body's circulatory system (see figure 3-3). We will enter the system at the inferior vena cava.

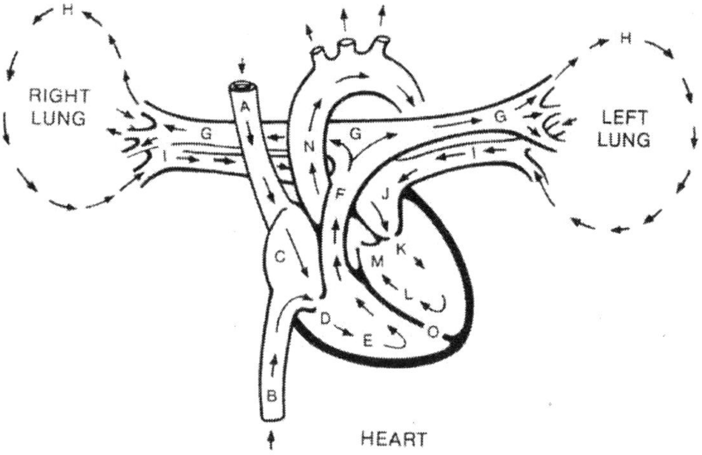

Direction of blood flow

A. Superior vena cava
B. Inferior vena cava
C. Right atrium
D. Tricuspid valve
E. Right ventricle
F. Pulmonary valve
G. Pulmonary arteries
H. Lungs
I. Pulmonary veins
J. Left ventricle
K. Mitral valve
L. Left ventricle
N. Aorta
O Interventricular septum

Figure 3-3. Blood flow to and from the heart. (Not drawn to scale; front view).

a. **Vena Cava.** There are two major blood veins that empty into the right atrium. The inferior vena cava carries oxygen-poor blood from the lower trunk and legs. The superior vena cava drains blood from the head and upper chest.

b. **Right Atrium.** The right atrium, the upper chamber of the right side of the heart, receives blood from the superior vena cava (blood from the upper body) and from the inferior vena cava (blood from the lower body). As the right atrium contracts, the rig ventricle relaxes. Contraction of the right atrium forces blood through the triscupid valve into the relaxed right ventricle. The triscupid valve is so formed that blood cannot flow back into the right atrium.

c. **Right Ventricle.** When the right ventricle is filled with blood, it receives an impulse from the sinoatrial (SA) node. This impulse causes the muscles of the right ventricle to contract. The contraction causes the inside of the ventricle (the space where the blood is) to become smaller. Increased pressure forces blood out of the ventricle and into the pulmonary artery. The pulmonary valve located at the beginning of the pulmonary artery keeps blood from flowing back into the right ventricle when the ventricle relaxes and returns to its normal size.

d. **Lungs (Pulmonary System).** The pulmonary artery divides into two arteries. One artery travels to the right lung while the other artery travels to the left lung. The arteries divide until they reach the capillary stage; the capillaries surround the alveoli (air sacs) of the lungs. There the oxygen-poor blood gets rid of its carbon dioxide and picks up oxygen from the air in the alveolus. The blood, now rich in oxygen, returns to the left atrium through the pulmonary veins.

e. **Left Atrium.** The left atrium receives blood from the lungs though two pulmonary veins. When the left ventricle relaxes after having contracted, blood flows from the left atrium into the left ventricle through the mitral valve. The mitral valve keeps blood from flowing back into the left atrium when the left ventricle contracts.

f. **Left Ventricle.** After the left ventricle is filled with oxygen-rich blood, it receives an impulse which causes it to contract and pump blood into the large artery called the aorta. When blood enters the aorta, it passes through the aortic valve. This valve keeps the blood from flowing back into the heart once the left ventricle relaxes.

g. **Body (Systemic System).** Arteries going to the head and upper body branch off the aorta. Two of these arteries (the right and left coronary arteries) supply the heart muscles with blood. After the aorta turns down, it divides into smaller arteries which go to the lower parts of the body. Arteries go to all parts of the body and divide into smaller blood vessels that eventually become capillaries. Blood in the capillaries give nutrients and oxygen to the cells and remove wastes. Capillaries then group to form veins that return blood to the right atrium. Before we leave the systemic circulatory system, though, let us take a brief look at the blood that flows to the intestines and to the kidneys.

(1) Intestines. Capillaries surrounding the intestines absorb fluids and nutrients from the intestines. Before returning to the heart, blood travels to the liver through the hepatic portal vein. In the liver, some of the nutrients are removed and stored for future use. The liver also removes bacteria and other types of unwanted substances from the blood. After passing through the liver, blood returns to the inferior vena cava through the hepatic vein.

(2) Kidneys. Some of the blood flows through the kidneys. The kidneys act as filters and remove most of the waste products contained in the blood. The major waste product removed is urea. The kidneys expel urea and other waste products in the form of urine.

Section II. GENERAL CONSIDERATIONS REGARDING CARDIAC ARREST

3-6. CARDIAC ARREST AND HEART ATTACK

It is important to understand the difference between cardiac arrest and a heart attack. Cardiac arrest (sudden death) is a result of the sudden and unexpected cessation of respiration and circulation. That is, the casualty stops breathing, and his heart stops beating. A heart attack is caused by a blockage of one or more of the coronary arteries (arteries which provide the heart muscles with oxygen-rich blood).

3-7. PRIMARY CAUSES OF CARDIAC ARREST

Cardiac arrest (cessation of the heartbeat) may occur for a number of reasons. Sixty percent of cardiac arrest cases occur as a result of cardiovascular diseases which include progression of myocardial infarction (death of myocardial cells due to an interrupted blood supply) and progression of heart rhythm disorders. Respiratory disease accounts for fifteen percent of cardiac arrest cases, and digestive and urogenital disease account for another seven percent of cardiac arrest cases. These miscellaneous cases make up the remaining three percent: hyperkalemia (abnormally high potassium concentration in the blood); electrical burns; metabolic disorders such as acidosis (disease resulting from accumulation of acid or depletion of alkaline in the blood and body tissues); trauma to the chest; pulmonary embolism (pulmonary artery or a branch being closed); intracerebral hemorrhage (bleeding in the cerebrum); and coronary artery spasm. When cardiac arrest occurs, oxygen is not circulated, and the body uses the oxygen stored in the vital organs in seconds.

3-8. MAJOR RISK FACTORS OF CARDIAC ARREST

a. **Statistics.** Statistics indicate that cardiac arrest is more likely to occur in these groups of individuals:

(1) Older persons.

(2) Individuals with a family history of arteriosclerosis (hardening of the arteries).

(3) Persons with hypertension (high blood pressure).

(4) Diabetes mellitus sufferers (body produces too little insulin, person very thirsty, and eats too much).

(5) Cigarette smokers.

(6) Those with elevated blood cholesterol.

(7) Persons with preexisting heart disease.

(8) Individuals who have premature ventricular complexes.

b. **Changing the Risk Factor.** Some risk factors cannot be changed: age, sex, race, and heredity. Other major risk factors, however, can be changed: cigarette smoking, hypertension, diabetes, and elevated cholesterol levels. The most important single cause of preventable death in the United States (US) is cigarette smoking. This habit begins and contributes to arteriosclerosis, myocardial infarction, and sudden death. Those who stop smoking return to the level of nonsmokers very rapidly. Hypertension (high arterial blood pressure) contributes to coronary artery disease, stroke, and heart failure. Control of hypertension makes a difference on whether or not a person survives cardiovascular problems. Research indicates that high total cholesterol levels increase the risk of coronary artery disease. Diet modification can lower the total cholesterol level thus decreasing the incidence of heart disease. A change to positive health behaviors can decrease the risk factors of cardiovascular problems.

3-9. MAJOR SIGNS OF CARDIAC ARREST

Cardiac arrest, the cessation of heartbeat, can occur for a variety of reasons. The major signs that the heart has stopped beating include sudden loss of consciousness, absence of pulse and respirations, cyanosis, and dilated pupils. Additionally, the dysrhythmias of cardiac arrest seen on a monitor include the following:

a. Ventricular fibrillation--an irregular and chaotic ventricular arrhythmia with a rapid rate and disorganized spread of impulses throughout the ventricular myocardium.

b. Ventricular tachycardia--abnormally rapid ventricular rate with broad QRS complexes and a rate between 100 and 200 beats per minute.

c. Asystole--absence of heartbeat.

d. Severe brady dysrhythmia--abnormally slow heartbeat with atrial and ventricular beats less than 60 beats per minute.

3-10. COMPONENTS OF THE DEFIBRILLATOR (LIFEPAK 5)

The defibrillator (Lifepack 5) is made up of these parts:

a. The electrocardiography monitor module (module and recorder).

b. A direct current (DC) defibrillator module with synchronizer. This piece of equipment has a charge time of 400 joules in 12.5 seconds and can deliver an electrical charge of 20, 30, 50, 100, 200 or 360 joules.

c. Patient cables.

d. A battery pack charger to recharge two batteries in 4 1/2 hours.

e. A nickel cadmium battery (the power source) which provides a minimum of twelve 360-joule discharges and 30 minutes of recorder use.

Section III. MAJOR MANAGEMENT TECHNIQUES OF CARDIAC ARREST

3-11. MONITORED CARDIAC ARREST

Monitored cardiac arrest is cardiac arrest (the cessation of heartbeats) that occurs when an electrocardiogram (EKG or ECG) is monitoring the casualty. Someone checking the monitor sees that the rhythm of the casualty's heart has changed to ventricular fibrillation. Ventricular fibrillation is a serious type of electrical failure in the heart. A ventricle receives extremely rapid, uncoordinated electrical signals that keep the heart from relaxing fully. When this happens in a ventricle, the affected part of the heart is unable to pump blood. An electric shock, if given in time, may cause the heart to beat again in normal rhythm. Follow this procedure to treat monitored cardiac arrest:

a. **Verify That There Is No Pulse.** Physically check for carotid pulse. Check the electrocardiogram equipment quickly to make sure that the problem is not just interference on the monitor due to cable or patient movement. If there is no pulse, do the next step.

b. **Perform Precardial Thump.** Using the fleshy part of your closed fist, deliver a thump eight to twelve inches above the sternum. This thump decreases the unreliability of the heart muscle and makes it less likely that the heart will start fibrillating. If this maneuver results in sinus rhythm (normal heart rhythm) with a pulse, proceed with lidocaine therapy. The dosage of lidocaine depends on the patient's condition. Usually, the dosage is I mg/kg with additional bolus injection of 0.5 mg/kg every 2 to 10 minutes, if needed, to a total dose of 3 mg/kg. The maintenance dosage is 2 to 4 mg.

c. **Defibrillate If Ventricular Fibrillation Persists.** Use an electrical charge of 200 joules. Give a nonsynchronized DC countershock. If 200 joules is unsuccessful, try 200 to 300 joules, then 360 joules, then CPR.

d. **Initiate Cardiopulmonary Resuscitation And Drug Therapy.** See Section IV and Section V of Lesson 1, Basic Cardiac Life Support.

e. **Procedure.** Proceed as you would for an unmonitored cardiac arrest. Refer to paragraph 3-12, UNMONITORED CARDIAC ARREST.

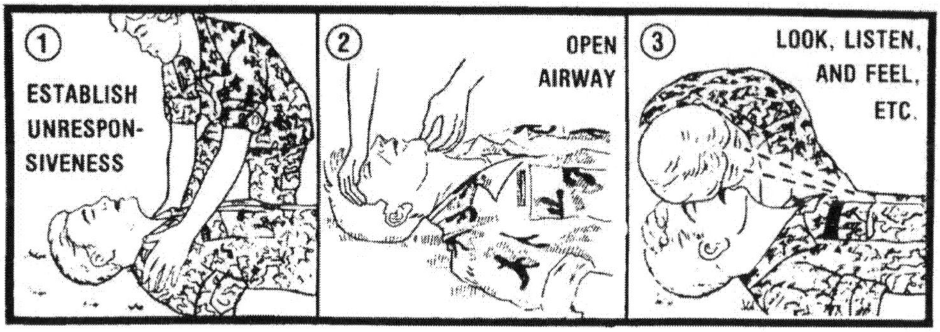

Figure 3-4. Cardiopulmonary resuscitation.

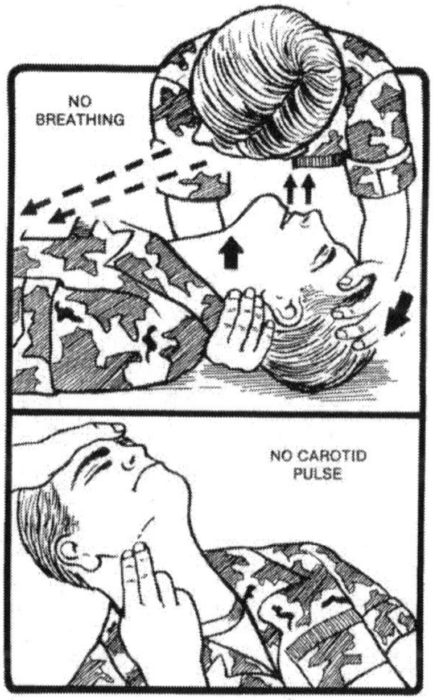

Figure 3-5. Basic cardiac life support.

3-12. **UNMONITORED CARDIAC ARREST**

Unmonitored cardiac arrest is cardiac arrest that occurs when the patient is not being monitored. Additionally, a defibrillator is not immediately available. Follow this procedure:

a. Initiate basic cardiac life support while a monitor defibrillator is being brought to the scene.

b. Take a "Quick-look" at the cardiac rhythm.

(1) Check to ensure that power is on and the oscilloscope (the instrument which shows electrical variations of the heartbeat on a screen) is functional (showing a line).

(2) Apply conductive media to paddles.

(3) Stop compressions.

(4) Use standard paddle placement to determine cardiac rhythm.

c. Defibrillate if ventricular fibrillation occurs.

(1) Set the electric charge 200 joules or according to panel instructions.

(2) Ensure that the paddles are firmly placed on the patient's chest with about 25 pounds of pressure.

(a) Place the negative paddle to the right of the upper sternum and below the right clavicle.

(b) Place the positive paddle below and to the left of the patient's left nipple.

(c) Apply downward pressure to each paddle.

(d) Remember that poor contact with the patient's skin will cause him to get burned when the machine is fired.

(e) Yell "Stand clear!" making sure that no one is directly or indirectly in contact with the patient.

(3) Administer a nonsynchronized countershock by pressing the discharge buttons on each paddle simultaneously.

(4) Release the thumb pressure from the discharge buttons.

(5) Check the cardiac rhythm.

(6) Check for a pulse.

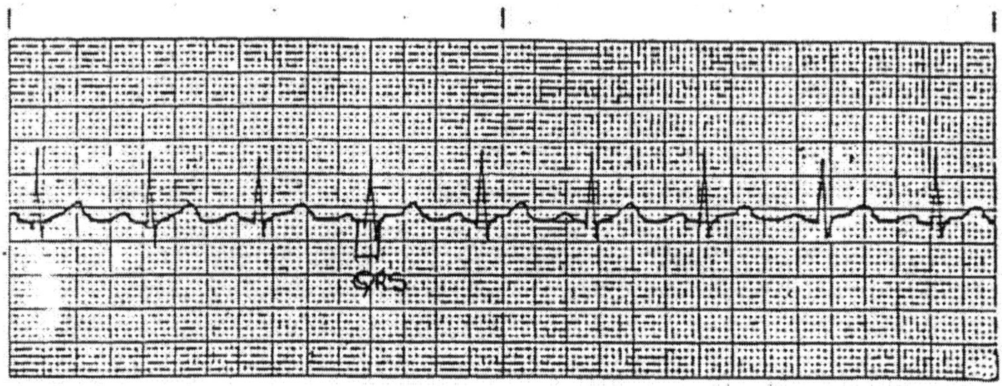

Figure 3-6. Normal cardiac rhythm.

(7) If the rhythm is adequate, check the carotid pulse to see if the pulse is associated with the rhythm shown on the oscilloscope. Also, check the vital signs and remain with the patient until he is evacuated.

d. If ventricular fibrillation continues, give a third countershock at 360 joules immediately.

e. If there is no pulse, this countershock has not been successful. Resume CPR.

f. Establish an effective airway. (Endotracheal intubation is preferable.)

g. Establish an intravenous (IV) line. (Two lines are preferable.)

h. Administer drug therapy as clinically indicated. Epinephrine (adrenalin) in a 1:10,000 solution in the dosage 0.5 to 1 mg may be injected intravenously and repeated at five minute intervals, if necessary. Give endotracheally if an IV line cannot be established quickly.

i. If ventricular fibrillation still continues, administer the third countershock. Use an energy load of not more than 360 joules. Stop CPR before the countershock and resume CPR after the countershock, if necessary.

j. Administer other drug therapy as clinically indicated. Include lidocaine (Xylocaine) 50 to 100 mg IV push.

CAUTION: Do not exceed 225 mgs of lidocaine.) Also, include bretylium tosylate (Bretylol) in the dosage 5 mg/kg IV bolus if lidocaine is ineffective.

k. If ventricular tachycardia (ventricles beating together but very fast) is seen with "Quick-look" paddles, follow this procedure:

(1) Administer lidocaine in the dosage 50 to 100 mg IV bolus.

(2) If the patient is coping with the rhythm, perform synchronized cardioversion with an electrical charge of 50 joules, a low energy charge. The object is to try to shock the ventricles into normal rhythm.

NOTE: Sedate the casualty who is awake if there is time.

(3) If synchronized cardioversion is ineffective, repeat cardioversion.

NOTE: These definitions are important to remember. Synchronized cardioversion is a timed electro shock delivered to a patient, the shock triggered by the R wave of the patient's electrocardiogram. Defibrillation is a non-timed electro shock delivered to a patient.

(4) Continue treatment as for unmonitored ventricular fibrillation, but cardiovert rather than defibrillate.

l. If asystole (absence of heartbeat) is seen with "Quick-look" paddles, follow this procedure:

(1) Begin/continue cardiopulmonary resuscitation.

(2) Insert an endotracheal tube or an esophageal airway for optimal ventilation.

(3) Start an IV infusion.

NOTE: Defibrillation is NOT used with asystole because there is no electrical activity in the heart to correct.

(4) Give 0.5 mg to 1 mg intravenously of epinephrine.

(5) Administer 1.0 mg of atropine intravenously. Repeat one time in 5 minutes.

(6) Repeat epinephrine at five minute intervals.

(7) In rare instances, a temporary pacemaker can be used to restore the paced rhythm of the heart.

m. If there is electromechanical dissociation (organized electrical activity without myocardial contraction) when the patient's cardiac rhythm is NOT correlated with his pulse, use these procedures:

(1) Administer CPR with optimal ventilation. Open the airway and blow into the patient's mouth to begin the process of restoring breathing and heartbeat.

(2) Administer epinephrine. The recommended dosage is 0.5 mg to 1.0 mg (5 to 10 ml of a 1:10,000 solution) given intravenously. Repeat every five minutes during resuscitative efforts. DO NOT administer epinephrine in the same intravenous line as alkaline solutions such as sodium bicarbonate.

n. If electromechanical dissociation persists, give additional doses of epinephrine at time intervals and as clinical judgment dictates.

NOTE: Previously, sodium bicarbonate was recommended in the treatment of cardiac arrest. Currently, there is controversy over this drug's benefit. Therefore, use sodium bicarbonate only after you have tried therapies such as defibrillation, cardiac compression, intubation, epinephrine, and antiarrhythmics have been tried without success.

o. The causes of electromechanical dissociation must be considered. Correctable causes include hypovolemia, cardiac tamponade, tension pneumothorax, hypoxemia, and acidosis. Less correctable cause of EMD include massive myocardial damage from miocardial infarction, prolonged ischemia during resuscitation, and pulmonary embolism.

SECTION IV. CARDIOVERSION

3-13. ATTACH THE PATIENT TO THE CARDIAC MONITOR

Follow this procedure:

a. Rub the electrode site with an alcohol pad to remove oil and dead tissue from the surface. (Shave hair if necessary.)

b. Apply conductive paste or gel to the electrodes and attach the electrodes to the chest.

CAUTION: Never use alcohol on electrodes. Alcohol could ignite and burn the patient.

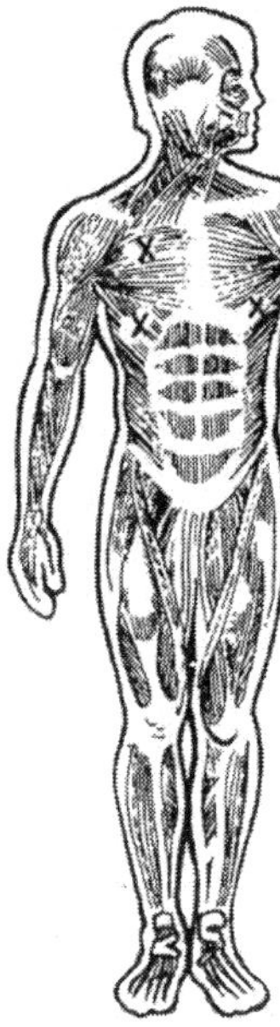

Figure 3-7. Electrode placement.

c. Use "Lead II" placement for the electrodes to measure the electrical output of the heart.

(1) Place the positive electrode below the left pectoral muscle.

(2) Place the negative electrode below the right clavicle.

(3) Place the ground electrode below the right pectoral muscle or below the left clavicle.

d. Attach the electrodes to the patient's monitoring cable.

3-14. PERFORM CARDIOVERSION PROCEDURE

Synchronized cardioversion is the use of the DC defibrillator to stop abnormal cardiac rhythms other than ventricular fibrillation. The procedure to follow is the same as for defibrillation with these exceptions:

a. The doctor may order diazepam (Valium) for a conscious patient.

b. The QRS complex on the monitor must be upright with maximum R-wave.

(1) P is a small positive deflection seen on the oscilloscope occurring right before Q. P represents the atria depolarization.

(2) Q is a negative (downward) deflection.

(3) R is the positive (upward) deflection and the highest point seen on the oscilloscope.

(4) S is a negative (downward) deflection seen on the oscilloscope.

(5) T is the positive deflection seen on the oscilloscope occurring after QRS complex. T represents the repolarization of the heart.

c. Switch on the synchronizer.

d. Yell, "Clear." before beginning.

e. Administer the initial shock of 200 joules. Some abnormal rhythms may be converted with shocks as low as 10 joules.

f. Press and hold the discharge buttons on the paddles until the defibrillator delivers the countershock.

g. If the initial countershock is not successful, use higher levels of energy on the next countershock.

h. If ventricular fibrillation occurs, follow this procedure:

(1) Turn off the synchronizer.

(2) Charge to between 200 to 300 joules.

(3) Defibrillate.

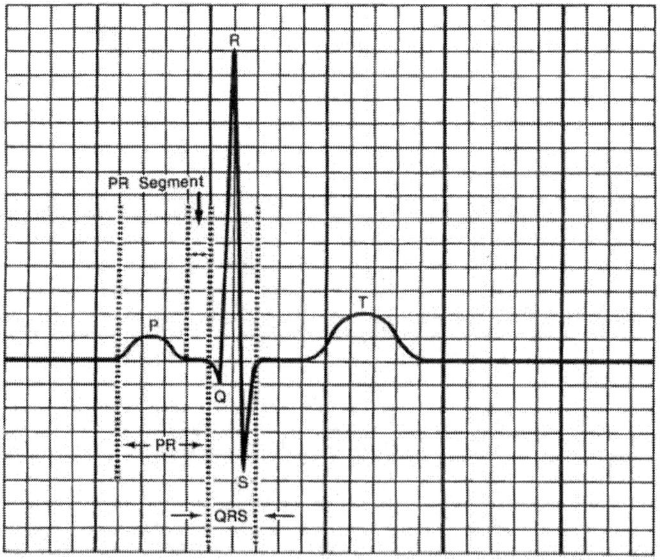

Figure 3-8. Electrocardiogram.

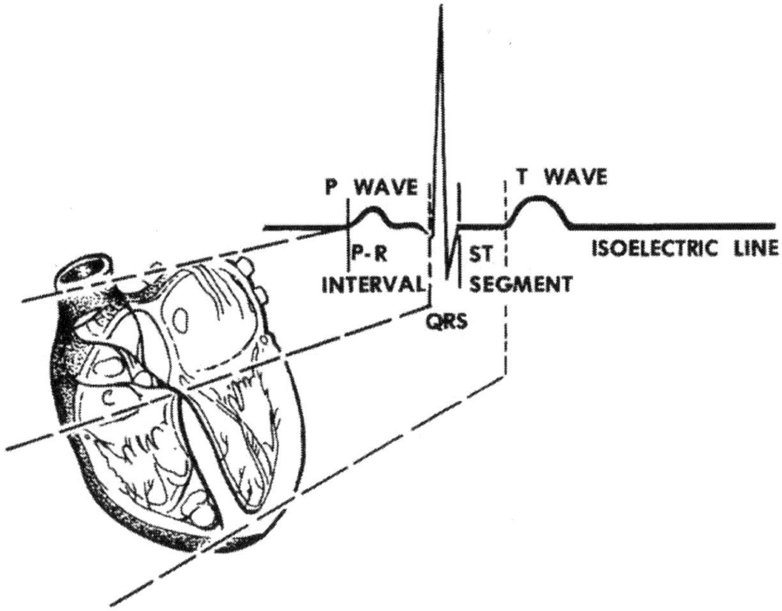

Figure 3-9. Electrocardiogram waves.

3-15. **CONCLUSION**

To prevent or treat a cardiac arrest effectively, you must first be able to recognize the problem and then apply the skills necessary for safe and effective management. Each situation presents a life or death series of decisions that must be varied to suit the patient. The guidelines you have learned in this lesson will be of valuable assistance to you in treating cardiac arrest.

Continue with Exercises

EXERCISES, LESSON 3

INSTRUCTIONS: The following exercises are to be answered by completing the incomplete statement or by writing the answer in the space provided at the end of the question. After you have completed all the exercises, turn to "Solutions to Exercises" at the end of the lesson and check your answers.

1. List the three primary causes of cardiac arrest.

   a. ______________________________.

   b. ______________________________.

   c. ______________________________.

2. List four groups of persons who are likely to have cardiac arrest.

   a. ______________________________.

   b. ______________________________.

   c. ______________________________.

   d. ______________________________.

3. Sudden loss of consciousness, absence of pulse and respirations, cyanosis, and dilated pupils are major signs that ______________________________.

4. The ECG monitoring has been started, but now the patient's heartbeat rhythm has deteriorated to ventricular fibrillation (monitored) or asystole. This is called ______________________________ cardiac arrest.

5. The patient is not being monitored and suffers cardiac arrest. This is called ______________________________ cardiac arrest.

6. You witness a cardiac arrest. The patient is being monitored on an ECG. Why should you verify pulseness?

____

____

7. These are the steps in managing monitored cardiac arrest. The steps are NOT in the order in which they would be performed. Choose the response which lists the steps in the order of performance.

   1. Initiate CPR.
   2. Perform precardial thump.
   3. Defibrillate if ventricular fibrillation persists.
   4. Verify pulselessness.
   5. Proceed as for unmonitored cardiac arrest.

   a 1,2,4,3,5.

   b. 4,2,3,1,5.

   c. 1,3,2,4,5.

   d. 4,1,5,3,2

8. The following statements are steps in managing unmonitored cardiac arrest. Fill in the blanks.

   a. Begin the procedure by initiating basic cardiac life support while __________ is being brought to the scene.

   b. Take a "Quick-look" at the ______________________________.

   c. If ventricular fibrillation occurs, ___________________________.

   d. If ventricular fibrillation continues, __________________________.

   e. If this is not successful, _________________________________.

   f. Next, set up ________________________________.

9. These are steps in getting ready to defibrillate a patient who is having ventricular fibrillation.

   a. Where do you place the negative paddle? ______________________________

   ____

   b. Where do you place the positive paddle? ______________________________

   ____

   c. If the paddles have poor contact with the patient's skin, what will happen when the machine fires?

   ____

   d. Before administering the countershock by pressing the discharge buttons on the machine, what should you do?

   ____

10. List one drug to be administered initially if drug therapy is indicated in

    unmonitored cardiac arrest. ______________________________________

11. List two drugs to be administered if the patient is having ventricular tachycardia after the third countershock in unmonitored cardiac arrest.

    a. ____.

    b. ____.

12. The "Quick-look" paddles indicate that the patient is suffering from ventricular tachycardia. You will follow these steps:

    a. Administer________________________________. (Name the drug.)

    b. Perform ____________________________________ cardioversion.

    c. Repeat cardioversion if __________________________ is ineffective.

    d. Continue as for unmonitored ventricular fibrillation, but ___________________ rather than defibrillate.

13. Why isn't defibrillation used on the patient with asystole?

____

14. What is electromechanical dissociation?

____

15. How is electromechanical dissociation determined?

______________________________.

16. What is cardioversion? ______________________________

____.

17. You are performing cardioversion on a patient with cardiac arrest and ventricular fibrillation occurs. List three things you must do immediately.

a. ______________________________.

b. ______________________________.

c. ______________________________.

18. The figure below shows an electrocardiogram representation of one heartbeat. Components of the electrocardiogram are marked with the letters A, B, C, D, E, F, G, and H. Opposite each letter write the letter name of the component as shown in the first blank line.

* A = P wave	* E = ______
* B = ______	* F = ______
* C = ______	* G = ______
* D = ______	* H = ______

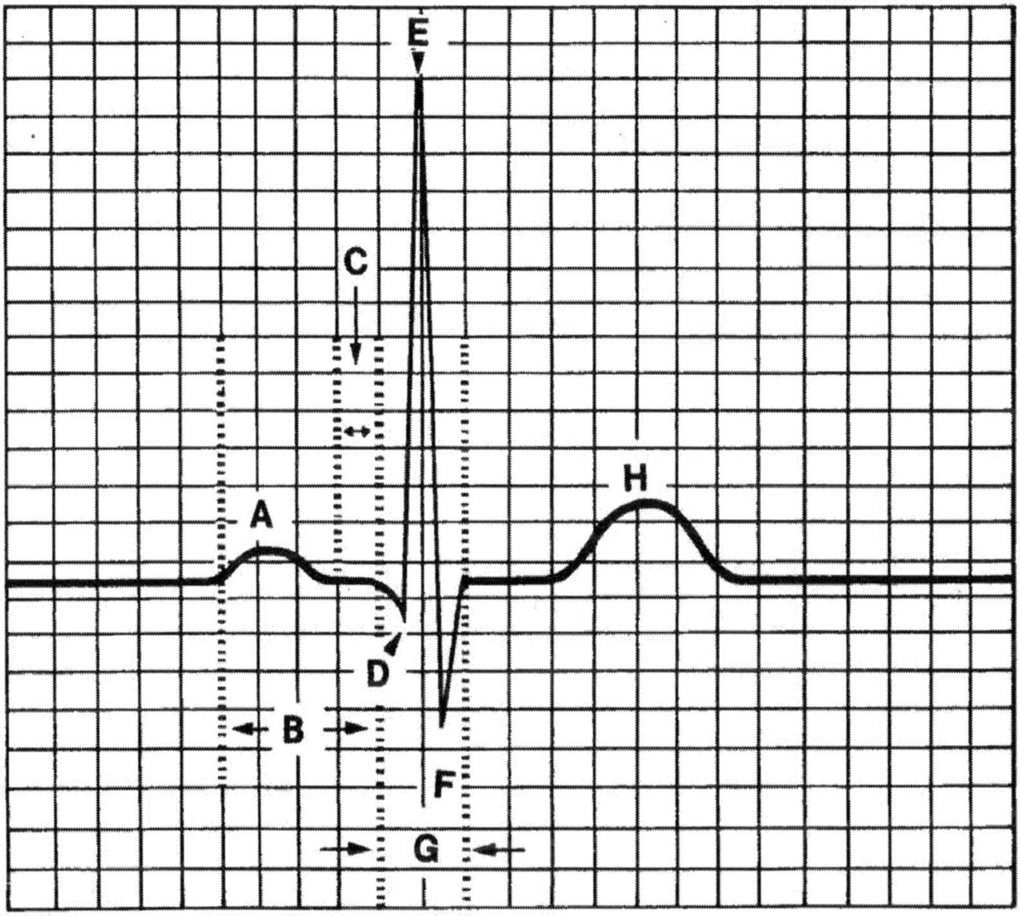

Check Your Answers on Next Page

SOLUTIONS TO EXERCISES, LESSON 3

1. You are correct if you listed any three of the following:

   . Results of cardiovascular diseases.
   . Respiratory diseases.
   . Central nervous system disease.
   . Digestive disease.
   . Urogenital disease.
   . Hyperkalemia.
   . Electrical burns.
   . Metabolic disorders.
   . Trauma to chest.
   . Pulmonary embolism.
   . Intracerebral hemorrhage.
   . Coronary artery spasm.

   (para 3-7)

2. You are correct if you listed any four of the following:

   . Older people.
   . People with family history of arteriosclerosis.
   . People with elevated blood cholesterol.
   . Patients with hypertension.
   . Diabetes mellitus sufferers.
   . Cigarette smokers.
   . Patients with preexisting heart disease.
   . People with premature ventricular complexes.

   (paras 3-8a and b)

3. The heart has stopped beating. (para 3-9)

4. Monitored. (para 3-11)

5. Unmonitored. (para 3-12)

6. Verify pulselessness to be sure there really is no pulse rather than just monitor interference because of cable or patient movement. para 3-11a)

7. b (paras 3-11a through e)

8. a. A monitor defibrillator.
   b. Cardiac rhythm.
   c. Defibrillate.
   d. Give a second countershock.
   e. Resume CPR.
   f. An effective airway. (para 3-12a through f)

9. a. Place the negative paddle to the right of the upper sternum and below the right clavicle.
   b. Place the positive paddle below and to the left of the patient's left nipple.
   c. The patient's skin will be burned.
   d. Yell "Stand clear!" and make sure no one has direct or indirect contact with the patient. (paras 3-12c(2)(a) through (e))

10. Epinephrine. (para 3-12h)

11. Lidocaine.
    Bretylium tosylate. (para 3-12j)

12. a. Lidocaine.
    b. Synchronized.
    c. Synchronized cardioversion.
    d. Cardiovert. (paras 3-12k(1) through (4))

13. Defibrillation is used when there is electrical activity in the heart. In asystole, there is no electrical activity in the heart; therefore, defibrillation is not used. (para 3-12l(3) NOTE)

14. Electromechanical dissociation is organized electrical activity without myocardial contraction. (para 3-12m)

15. Electromechanical dissociation is determined by correlating the cardiac rhythm to the patient's pulse. (para 3-12m)

16. Cardioversion is the use of the defibrillator to end abnormal cardiac rhythms, other than ventricular fibrillation. (para 3-14)

17. Turn off the synchronizer.
    Charge to between 200 to 300 joules.
    Begin defibrillation procedures. (paras 3-14h(1) through (3))

18. A = P wave   E = R wave

    B = P-R   F = S wave

    C = PR segment   G = QRS complex

    D = Q wave   H = T wave

    (paras 3-14b(1) through (5) and figure 3-9)

End of Lesson 3